P. Dawson W. Clauß (Hrsg.)

D0547713

Contrast Media in Practice

With 42 Figures and 18 Tables

Springer-Verlag
Berlin Heidelberg New York
London Paris Tokyo
Hong Kong Barcelona
Budapest

Dr. Peter Dawson
Department of Radiology
Hammersmith Hospital
Ducane Road, London W12 OHS
United Kingdom

Dr. Wolfram Clauß
Schering AG, Klinische Entwicklung Diagnostika
13342 Berlin

© Coverphotos: Pictor International

ISBN 3-540-57187-6 Springer-Verlag Berlin Heidelberg New York
ISBN 0-387-57187-6 Springer-Verlag New York Heidelberg Berlin

Library of Congress Cataloging-in-Publication Data

Contrast media in practice / P. Dawson, W. Clauss, (hrsg.)
    p. cm.
  ISBN 0-387-57187-6 (U.S.)
  1. Contrast media.   I. Dawson, Peter H.   II. Clauss, W.
(Wolfram), 1940–   .
RC78.7.C65C665   1993
616.07′54--dc20

© Springer-Verlag Berlin Heidelberg 1994
Printed in Germany

Printing and bookbinding: Druckhaus Beltz, 69502 Hemsbach
Typesetting: Cicero Lasersatz, 86167 Augsburg, Germany
21/3145-543210 – Printed on acid-free paper

Contents

4 Determination of Risk Factors Regarding the Administration of Contrast Media

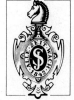

5 Prophylactic Measures

8 Adverse Reactions and Their Pathophysiology and Management

10 Contrast Media for Magnetic Resonance Imaging and Ultrasound

Contributors

Adam, A., Prof., Dept. of Radiology, Guy's Hospital, London Bridge,
London SE1 9 RT, UK

Alhassan, A., Dr., Schering AG, Arzneimittelsicherheit,
Müllerstraße 170–178, 13342 Berlin, Germany

Andrew, E., Dr., Nycomed AS Imaging, Slemdalsveien 37, 0301 Oslo 3,
Norway

Bassir, C., Dr., Univ.-Klinikum Rudolf Virchow, FUB, Pädiatrische
Radiologie, KAVH, Heubnerweg 6, 12487 Berlin, Germany

Bohn, H. P., Dr., Nycomed AS Imaging, Slemdalsveien 37, 0301 Oslo 3,
Norway

Brasch, Robert C., Prof., University of California, Department of
Radiology, Contrast Media Laboratory, Third and Parnassus Street,
San Francisco, CA 94143, USA.

Clauß, Wolfram, Dr., Schering AG, Klinische Entwicklung Diagnostika,
Müllerstraße 170–178, 13342 Berlin, Germany

Davies, Peter, Dr., F.R.C.R., Department of Radiology, City Hospital,
Nottingham, UK

Dawson, Peter, Dr., Dept. of Radiology, Univ. of London, Royal
Postgraduate Medical School, Hammersmith Hospital, Ducane Road,
London W12 OHS, UK

Dickerhoff, Roswitha, Dr., Kinderklinik, St. Augustin,
Arnold-Janssen-Straße 29, 53757 St. Augustin, Germany

Dihlmann, W., Prof., Röntgeninstitut, Allgemeines Krankenhaus Barmbek,
Rübenkamp 148, 22307 Hamburg, Germany

Dinger, J. C., Dr., Schering AG, GCP Methologie,
Müllerstraße 170–178, 13353 Berlin, Germany

Glöbel, B., Prof. Dr., Univ.-Kliniken des Saarlandes, Abteilung
Medizintechnik und Strahlenschutz, 66424 Homburg, Germany

Grainger, Ronald G., Prof., Royal Hallamshire Hospital,
Department of Radiology, Glossop Road, Sheffield S10 2JF, UK

Günzel, P., Dr., Schering AG, Experimentelle Toxikologie,
Müllerstraße 170–178, 13342 Berlin, Germany

Gulbrandsen, Trygve, Dr., Nycomed AS Imaging, Slemdalsveien 37,
0301 Oslo 3, Norway

Hagen, Bernd, Dr., Martin-Luther-Krankenhaus, Röntgen- und
Strahlenabteilung, Caspar-Theyss-Straße 27–31, 14194 Berlin, Germany

Heep, Josef, Prof., Josefskrankenhaus, Gynäkologische Abteilung,
Landhausstraße 25, 69115 Heidelberg, Germany

Hering, L., Dr., Röntgeninstitut, Allgemeines Krankenhaus Barmbek,
Rübenkamp 148, 22307 Hamburg, Germany

Herrmann, Dirk, Dr., Schering AG, Müllerstraße 170–178, 13342 Berlin,
Germany

Imhof, H., Prof., Zentrales Inst. für Radiodiagnostik, Allgemeines
Krankenhaus Wien, Lazarettgasse 14, 1090 Wien, Austria

Katayama, Hitoshi, Prof., Department of Radiology, Juntendo University,
Hongo 3-1-3, Brunkyo-ku, Tokyo 113, Japan

Kaufmann, Herbert J., Prof., Schwerinstraße 14, 10783 Berlin, Germany

Krause, Werner, Dr., Schering AG, Forschung Röntgenkontrastmittel,
Müllerstraße 170–178, 13342 Berlin, Germany

Krestin, G., Dr., Med. Einrichtungen d. Univ., Radiologische Inst.
und Poliklinik, Joseph-Stelzmann-Straße 9, 50931 Köln, Germany

Laerum, Frode, Prof., Section for Experimental Radiology,
Department of Diagnostic Radiology, Rikshospitalet,
0027 Oslo 1, Norway

Maurer, H.-J., Prof., Obere Flurstraße 11, 88131 Lindau-Bodolz, Germany

Niendorf, Hans-Peter, Dr., Schering AG, Klinische Entwicklung
Diagnostika, Müllerstraße 170–178, 13342 Berlin, Germany

Papassotiriou, V., Dr., Wenckebach-Krankenhaus, Röntgenabteilung,
Wenckebachstraße 23, 12099 Berlin, Germany

Richards, David, Dr., Department of Radiology, Middlesex Hospital, Mortimer Street, London W1N 8AA, UK

Rödl, W., Prof., Klinikum Weiden, Abteilung Radiologische Diagnostik, 92637 Weiden, Germany

Romaniuk, Paul, Prof., Inst. für Kardiovaskuläre Diagnostik, Charite-Humboldt-Universität, Schumannstraße 20–21, 10117 Berlin, Germany

Sage, Michael R., Prof., Dept. of Radiology, The Flinders University of South Australia, Flinders Medical Centre, Bedford Park, South Australia 5042, Australia

Scherberich, J. E., Dr., Klinikum der J.-W.-Goethe-Universität, Zentrum der Inneren Medizin, Theodor-Stern-Kai 7, 60596 Frankfurt, Germany

Schlief, Reinhard, Dr., Schering AG, Klinische Entwicklung Diagnostika, Müllerstraße 170–178, 13342 Berlin, Germany

Schöbel, Christel, Dr., Schering AG, Experimentelle Toxikologie, Müllerstraße 170–178, 13342 Berlin, Germany

Schürmann, R., Dr., Schering AG, Klinische Entwicklung Diagnostika, Müllerstraße 170–178, 13342 Berlin, Germany

Schuhmann-Gampieri, Gabriele, Dr., Schering AG, Forschung Röntgenkontrastmittel, Müllerstraße 170–178, 13342 Berlin, Germany

Skalpe, I. O., Prof., Rikshospitalet, Röntgen-Radium-Avd., Pilestredet 32, 0027 Oslo 1, Norway

Spann, W., Prof., Ludwig-Maximilians-Univ., Fachbereich Medizin, Bavariastraße 19, 80336 München, Germany

Speck, Ulrich, Prof., Schering AG, Diagnostika Forschung, Müllerstraße 170–178, 13342 Berlin, Germany

Strickland, Nicola Hilary, Dr., Dept. of Radiology, Royal Postgraduate Medical School, Hammersmith Hospital, Ducane Road, London W12 OHS, UK

Taenzer, V., Prof., Krankenhaus Moabit, Röntgenabteilung, Turmstraße 21, 10559 Berlin, Germany

Tauber, R., Prof., Allgemeines Krankenhaus Barmbek, Urologische Abteilung, Rübenkamp 148, 22307 Hamburg, Germany

Thelen, Manfred, Prof., Klinikum der Johannes-Gutenberg-Universität,
  Institut für Klinische Strahlenkunde, Langenbeckstraße 1, 55131 Mainz,
  Germany

Thron, A., Prof., Neurologische Klinik der RWTH,
  Abteilung Neuroradiologie, Pauwellsstraße, 52074 Aachen, Germany

Vergesslich, Klara, Dr., Universitätskinderklinik Wien,
  Währinger Gürtel 18–20, 1090 Wien, Austria

Weissleder, H., Prof., Kreiskrankenhaus, Abt. für Röntgendiagnostik,
  Gartenstraße 40, 70312 Emmendingen, Germany

Wisser, Gregor, Dr., Klinikum der Johannes-Gutenberg-Universität,
  Klinik für Anästhesiologie, Langenbeckstraße 1, 55131 Mainz, Germany

Wolden, Brit, Dr., Nycomed AS Imaging, Slęmdalsveien 37, 0301 Oslo 3,
  Norway

Zuckert, Dieter, Dr., Kissinger-Straße 57, 14199 Berlin, Germany

CHAPTER 1

General Fundamentals

1.1 A Historical Overview of the Development of Contrast Media for Diagnostic Imaging Procedures in Radiology

H. J. Maurer and *W. Clauss*

In diagnostic imaging, a distinction is made between negative X-ray (air, O_2, CO_2), positive X-ray (barium $BaSO_4$; iodine, I), paramagnetic, and ultrasonographic contrast media (CM). Barium sulphate ($BaSO_4$) had already been used in 1896 for investigations on peristalsis, but it was forgotten again once the study was concluded. It was only about a decade later that $BaSO_4$, "newly" developed by the pharmacist and final-year medical student Fritz Munk, was introduced into X-ray investigations of the gastrointestinal tract as the so-called Rieder meal (barium mixed with gruel). It has been able to maintain its predominant position up to the present day, albeit with certain modifications such as taste corrigents and changes in density and particle size, though occasionally it is replaced by tri-iodinated ionic or nonionic X-ray CM, which are used, for example, in suspected fistulae, ileus, or for an array of purposes in children.

Iodine was recognized as an X-ray-absorber, i. e., as a positive X-ray CM, as early as 1896 (Haschek and Lindenthal), but the implications of this were not immediately recognized. The iodized oil Lipiodol was successfully introduced into myelography by Sicard as the first usable X-ray CM other than air in 1921. This oily X-ray CM, used at the same time for bronchography, and later for hysterosalpingography, pyelography, pyeloscopy, and, above all, lymphography, was poorly absorbed, largely because of its molecular size; this often led to foreign-body granulomata. Because of the occurrence of pulmonary and peripheral fat microemboli, oily X-ray CM are hardly ever indicated today, except in such conditions as destructive chronic pulmonary diseases and pulmonary hypertension. Sicard and Jacobaeus also used Lipiodol for ventriculography, but the complications arising were one reason why this not become an established procedure.

Water-soluble X-ray CM are subdivided into renal and biliary X-ray CM, which are chiefly distinguished by the ways in which they bind to proteins. In contrast to uroangiographic media, which are excreted by the kidney after passive glomerular filtration, cholegraphic agents reach the liver only after binding to serum proteins and are excreted via the gallbladder after metabolism. Since toxicity increases along with increasing protein binding, the objective must be to develop renal X-ray CM with minimal protein binding and biliary X-ray CM with the lowest possible degree of protein binding.

Oral cholecystography, still occasionally used today despite the good results of ultrasonography (US), allows visualization of the gallbladder if the small intestine absorbs the CM; it cannot, however, do the same for the bile ducts. If the whole of the biliary system, i. e., the intra- and extrahepatic biliary tree including the gallbladder, must be visualized, this should be attempted using a rapid-infusion cholecystocholangiography, possibly in conjunction with tomography or thick-section tomography ("zonography") and/or computed tomography (CT).

Oral Biliary X-Ray Contrast Media

In 1909, it was shown that phenoltetrachlorophthalein is excreted by the gallbladder. This effect was then used for testing liver function from 1916 into the 1950s. In 1923, the gallbladder was demonstrated using orally administered halogenated phenolphthalein. In 1924 iodophthalein sodium (Iodtetragnost) was put on the market and then in 1940 Dohrn and Diedrich developed iodoalphionic acid (Biliselectan), which had only half the toxicity of iodophthalein sodium. The development of a series of oral cholecystographic agents such as sodium ipodate (Biloptin) then followed. These new agents were all based on the same basic structure, but with different side chains, and were characterized by their better tolerability.

Biliary Intravenous X-Ray Contrast Media

While attempting to synthesize a better renal X-ray CM, Priewe administered intravenously a compound consisting of two molecules of acetrizoate connected by an aliphatic chain, and was surprised to find excretion occurring via the liver and biliary system. From this, Langecker, Hawart and Junkmann [5] developed the first hepatic-biliary X-ray CM, iodipamide (adipiodone; Biligrafin); in 1953, Frommhold introduced it into routine practice. Due to the relatively high toxicity of Biligrafin and similar preparations, further substances were subsequently synthesized and developed which, ultimately, led to iotroxic acid (Biliscopin), a medium which displays goodle tolerability when used in the brief-infusion cholecystocholangiogram.

Renal X-Ray Contrast Media

Even though iodine was recognized very early as a positive X-ray CM (1896), it still took about 30 years for a clinically acceptable X-ray CM to be developed. The procedure that Berberich and Hirsch as well as Moniz chose, namely, to administer bromide compounds (Sr, Br, LiB_r, KB_r, NaB_r) intravenously and intraarterially in order to image the blood vessels, resulted in some cases in technically successful arteriographies and phlebographies. The inadequate vessel demonstration and the severe intolerance reactions, especially following intraarterial administration, prompted Moniz to try sodium iodide, which Osborne, Sutherland, Scholl [8] and Roundtree had already used for intravenous urography in 1923. In spite of the high toxicity of the 25% sodium iodide solution used, the good contrast-enhancing properties of iodine were demonstrated. These are chiefly the result of the high mass absorption coefficient that iodine possesses at the wavelengths used in diagnostic radiology.

In a completely different context, in 1925, Binz and Räth [2] synthesized various pyridine compounds, some of which also contained iodine. Swick [11], investigated a series of these pyridines in 1928 and 1929, first with L. Lichtwitz (City Hospital of Altona, Hamburg, Germany) and later with A. von Lichtenberg (St. Hedwig's Hospital, Berlin, Germany) [6]. In conjunction with Schering AG, he then developed Selectan Neutral in 1929, which was very quickly supplemented by Uroselectan (1 iodine atom) and Uroselectan B (2 iodine atoms). At about the same time (1930), Bronner, Hecht and Schüller at Bayer AG developed Abrodil (methiodal sodium – iodomethanesulfonic acid as the sodium salt) and Per-Abrodil (iodopyracet – 3,5-iodo-4-pyridone-N-acetic acid). The diiodinated X-ray CM Uroselectan and Per-Abrodil provided adequate imaging of the efferent urinary tract and of the blood vessels with satisfactory tolerability; they were used for almost 20 years in diagnostic radiology.

In 1929, Moniz [7] introduced a thorium-dioxide suspension for cerebral angiography; it provided excellent contrast and was very well tolerated. However, a great proportion of the thorium is stored in the reticuloendothelial system and leads, because of its radioactivity, to the formation of benign tumours, which in time become malignant. In extravascular injections, considerable fibrosis develops, which may compress the vessel and may also become malignant. Even though these serious complications were known in 1942, thorium dioxide continued to be used, although increasingly less often, into the 1950s.

At the beginning of the 1950s, the change was made from diiodinated pyridine derivatives to benzene derivatives with three substituted iodine atoms, i.e., triiodinated benzoic acid derivatives. Hydrophilic side groups and the meglumine cation improved the tolerability of the ionic CM considerably, while the third iodine atom bound to the molecule led to higher contrast density.

The development of these triiodinated X-ray CM was initiated by Wallingford's synthesis [12] of acetrizoate sodium (Urokon Sodium, Mallinckrodt, 1950). Diedrich (Schering) and chemists at Sterling-Winthrop simultaneously succeeded in making a decisive further improvement in tolerance by synthesizing meglumine diatrizoate (Urografin and Hypaque, 1954). By starting with meglumine diatrizoate and varying the side chains, the following preparations were then developed: metrizoic acid (Isopaque, 1962), iothalamic acid (Conray, 1962), iodamide (Uromiro, 1965), ioxitalamic acid

(Telebrix, 1972) and ioglicic acid (Rayvist, 1978). For more than 30 years, these X-ray CM formed the basis for diagnostic studies of the blood vessels, the renal tract, and various body cavities. They are still used today, although primarily intravenously. What they have in common are their dissociation into anions and cations (as ionic X-ray CM) and their consequent high osmotic pressure (up to seven times that of blood). Almen [1] was the first at the end of the 1960s to recognize the decisive role that hyperosmolality and electrical charge play in triggering certain side effects of ionic X-ray CM. His suggestion of replacing the ionic carboxyl radical in the triiodinated benzoic-acid derivatives with a nondissociating group and to guarantee the required water solubility by means of substituting hydrophilic OH groups represented the birth of nonionic X-ray CM.

The osmolality, more closely approaching that of the blood, and the lack of electrical charge clearly improved tolerability. Amipaque was chiefly used for myelography and occasionally peripheral angiography; nevertheless, it still had to be made up into solution immediately prior to use. The introduction of nonionic triiodinated X-ray CM in ready-to-use form, such as iohexol (Omnipaque), iopamidol (Solutrast, Niopam, Isovue, Iopamiron), iopromide (Ultravist), ioversol (Optiray) and iopentol (Imagopaque), made the use of nonionic X-ray CM easier and thus promoted such use. The effort to achieve similarly favourable results by using the ionic dimer ioxaglic acid (Hexabrix) was, however, not quite as successful. Nonionic X-ray CM can be used in all regions of the body, except for the biliary and lymphatic systems.

Numerous publications based on clinically monitored comparative studies have demonstrated the significantly lower rates of mild and moderate side effects that nonionic X-ray CM have in comparison to ionic ones. However, as yet, only three large-scale, multicentre studies have been carried out with the goal of differentiating X-ray CM in terms of the severe reactions they all, rarely, trigger. Independent of statistical design, the results of all three studies attest to the reduced risk of severe, life-threatening reactions occurring when nonionic X-ray CM are used. This reduction in risk varies from a factor of 1:2 to 1:10, depending upon the type and degree of prior impairment of the patient [4, 9, 10].

The synthesis of the hexaiodinated nonionic dimers iotralan (Isovist), iodecol and iodixanol (Visipaque) represents the most recent advance in X-ray CM development. The osmolality of these media in all concentrations matches that of circulating blood; indeed, their osmolality has to be adjusted upwards to achieve this. It is possible to reduce significantly the neurotoxic symptoms associated with myelography by using iotrolan, which is already commercially available. The suitability for intravascular use of the non-ionic dimers is currently being tested in comparative clinical studies.

The attempt to replace the contrast-enhancing element, iodine, with lithium, widely used in psychiatry, had to be abandoned after animal experiments in spite of the good contrast it provided, since considerable cystic degeneration of the kidneys was observed.

Negative CM such as air, O_2 and CO_2 do not absorb X-rays as strongly as body tissues do; this allows one to achieve a negative contrast effect in certain body cavities. Very early, prior to US and CT use was made of air in imaging the kidney, ureter and bladder. Following presacral insufflation, air, O_2 and CO_2 also allowed the imaging of retroperitoneal and mediastinal structures, especially in combination with tomography. In addition, CO_2 was used both experimentally and clinically for angiocardiography and aortoarteriography, in order to avoid administering iodinated X-ray CM to patients at risk. Difficulties in its administration and often inadequate contrast have hindered its routine use.

Negative CM were primarily administered in ventriculography and ascending lumbar or basal cisternography. However, their use was first limited by the introduction of cerebral angiography; then, later, CT and, today, magnetic resonance imaging (MRI), have completely superceded them. In the same way, the use of pneumomyelography was considerably reduced on the introduction of Lipiodol-based myelography, later replaced by di- and triiodinated ionic X-ray CM. Today, myelography is performed exclusively using nonionic monomeric and dimeric X-ray CM that are eliminated via the urine.

Summary

Seen as a whole, the history of iodinated X-ray CM represents a successful and happy example of collaboration between the chemical-pharmaceutical industry and clinicians. As a result, diagnostic radiology has available very well tolerated, nonionic X-ray CM for all applications.

In order to complete the picture, it should be mentioned that for MRI and US, paramagnetic CM (such as Gd-DTPA and Gd-DOTA) and a CM based on microbubbles, respectively, have been developed and made commercially available. The use of these CM has made it possible to increase considerably the sensitivity and specificity of these diagnostic procedures.

References

1. Almén T (1969) Contrast agent design. Some aspects of the synthesis of water-soluble agents of low osmolality. J Theor Biol 24:216–226
2. Binz A, Räth A, von Lichtenberg A (1931) The chemistry of proselectan. Z Urol 25:297–301
3. Grainger RG (1982) Intravascular contrast media – the past, the present and the future. Br J Radiol 55:1–18
4. Katayama H, Yamaguchi K, Kozuka T, Takashima T, Seez P, Matsuura K (1990) Adverse reactions to ionic and nonionic contrast media. A report from the Japanese Committee on the Safety of Contrast Media. Radiology 175:621–628
5. Langecker H, Harwart A, Junkmann K (1954) 3,5-Diacetylamino-2,4,6-triiodbenzoesäure als Röntgenkontrastmittel. Naunyn-Schmiedebergs Arch Exp Pathol 222:584–590
6. Lichtenberg A von, Swick M (1929) Klinische Prüfung des Uroselectans. Klin Wochenschr 8:2089–2091

7. Moniz E (1934) L'angiographie cérébrale. Masson, Paris
8. Osborne ED, Sutherland CG, Scholl AF, Rowntree LG (1923) Roentgenography of urinary tract during excretion of sodium iodide. JAMA 80:368–373
9. Palmer FJ (1988) The RACR survey of intravenous contrast media reactions: final report. Austral Radiol 32:426–428
10. Schrott KM, Behrends B, Clauß W, Kaufmann J, Lehnert J (1986) Iohexol in der Ausscheidungsurographie: Ergebnisse des Drug monitorings. Fortschr Med 7:53–156
11. Swick M (1929) Darstellung der Niere und Harnwege im Röntgenbild durch intra-venöse Einbringung eines neuen Kontraststoffes, des Uroselectans. Klin Wochenschr 8:2087–2089
12. Wallingford VH (1953) The development of organic iodide compounds as X-ray contrast media. J Am Pharmacol Assoc (Sci Ed) 42:721–728

1.2 Chemistry of X-Ray Contrast Media

T. Gulbrandsen

Introduction

Obviously, the function of X-ray CM is to opacify an organ or portion of the body to X-rays. X-rays interact with, and are absorbed by, electrons and this absorption is known to be approximately proportional to the atomic number to the power of three. Thus, any heavy atom packed into a biologically acceptable environment is a potential candidate as an X-ray CM. In modern history, iodine has been the only heavy atom possessing all the chemical properties necessary for inclusion in suitable CM for intravascular and intrathecal use.

Physicochemical Properties

Water Solubility

Due to the rather insensitive detection methods for X-rays, iodine must be introduced into the body part to be examined at a concentration of at least 100 mg/ml. In vascular applications an immediate dilution with blood occurs and, to give sufficient contrast, quite high concentrations of iodine must be injected. It is essential to design CM with extremely high aqueous solubility, without there being any danger of crystal formation in the vials or syringes, or in the body. The following chemical principles can be applied to improve the solubility in water:
– Ionic groups, i.e. salts
– Hydroxyl groups (more than three) and other hydrophilic groups.
– High number of structural isomers.

Viscosity

The higher the viscosity of the solution, the longer it will take for the CM to be diluted by blood to diagnostically unuseful concentrations. However, in clinical practice viscosity limits the injection rate, particularly when injecting through a catheter. Thus, there are optimal viscosities for CM that vary with the clinical indication. Factors influencing the viscosity of CM solutions are:
– The number of hydroxyl groups and the size and geometry of substituent groups
– The molecular weight of the CM
– The temperature of the solution.

In fact, by heating the CM solution to body temperature, viscosity may be decreased by 50%. Injection at body temperature is beneficial as regards pharmacological effects as well, particularly in cardiac use.

Osmolality

Parenteral injections should have an osmolality as close to that of body fluids as possible. Since the osmolality of a solution is directly proportional to the number of dissolved particles (molecules, ions) the osmolality of CM solutions can be decreased by increasing the number of iodine atoms per dissolved particle (Table 1.2.1).

Table 1.2.1. Osmolality in the four categories of contrast media

Compound	Iodine atoms	Particles	Ratio
Ionic monomers	3	2	1.5
Nonionic monomers	3	1	3.0
Ionic dimers	6	2	3.0
Nonionic dimers	6	1	6.0

In the present state of the art, CM can be classified under four categories:
1. Ionic monomers, characterized by one triiodobenzene ring containing one carboxyl group.
   Examples: Metrizoate (Isopaque), diatrizoate (Hypaque)
2. Ionic monoacid dimers, characterized by two triiodobenzene rings linked together by a carbon-chain bridge, with one of the triiodo-benzene groups carrying a carboxyl group.
   Example: Ioxaglate (Hexabrix)
3. Nonionic monomers, characterized by one triiodobenzene ring carrying more than three hydroxyl groups, with no carboxyl or other ionizing groups.

Examples: iohexol (Omnipaque), iopamidol (Iopamiro, Niopam, Isovue), iopromide (Ultravist), ioversol (Optiray), iopentol (Imagopaque)
4. Nonionic dimers, characterized by two triiodobenzene rings linked together by a carbon-chain bridge, carrying several hydroxyl groups and without ionizing groups.
Examples: iodixanol (Visipaque), iotrolan (Isovist).

A further step toward in the ultimate goal in the development of more low-osmolar compounds has been made with iodixanol and iotrolan nonionic dimers, which currently are the only X-ray CM forming isotonic solutions above 300 mg I/ml.

Distribution of Hydrophilic Substituents

Toxicity of a chemical substance is largely caused by its interactions with proteins, membranes, etc. in the body. It is generally accepted that lipophilic groups in a molecule interact more readily with biomolecules than hydrophilic groups. Thus, it can be deduced that a molecule with optimal biological acceptance should not only be highly hydrophilic, but should also have its hydrophilic substituents evenly distributed around its surface. The higher tolerance of iohexol compared to that of metrizamide may be partly explained by the more even distribution of hydroxyl groups around the iohexol molecule, metrizamide being divided into a hydrophilic part (the glucosamine) and a lipophilic part (the iodinated aromatic ring) (Fig. 1.2.1).

It must be kept in mind that the molecules are not planar, but roughly globular shapes in three-dimensional space.

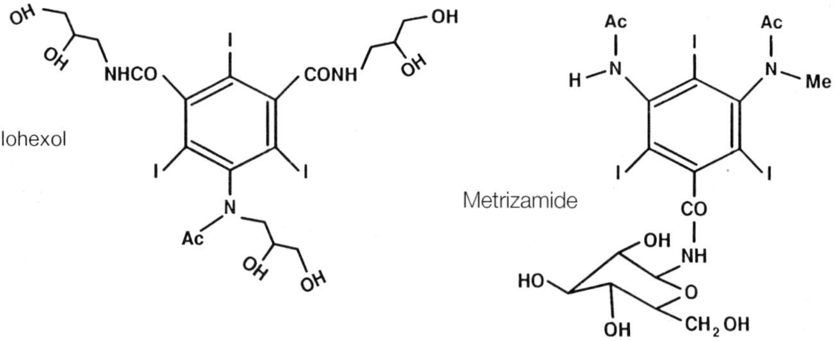

Fig. 1.2.1. Structural formulae of iohexol and metrizamide

Chemical Stability

CM are stable for years when kept at room temperature, protected from light. The stability of some media has also been documented at 40 °C. The first sign of degradation of a X-ray CM is the liberation of iodide ions into the solution. This degradation reaction is facilitated by heat, exposure to light or contamination with traces of copper ions. For this reason, contrast solutions contain ethylenediaminetetracetic acid (EDTA), which forms a stable complex with copper.

Synthesis

The synthesis of ionic CM is quite simply accomplished using three- or four-step methods from industrially available 3,5-dinitrobenzoic acid or 5-nitro-isophthalic acid. 3,5-Dinitrobenzoic acid is transformed into 3,5-diamino-benzoic acid by catalytic hydrogenation, followed by iodination with iodine chloride (or sodium iodine dichloride in aqueous solution), and transformed further into diatrizoic acid by acetylation of the amino groups with acetic anhydride (Fig. 1.2.2).

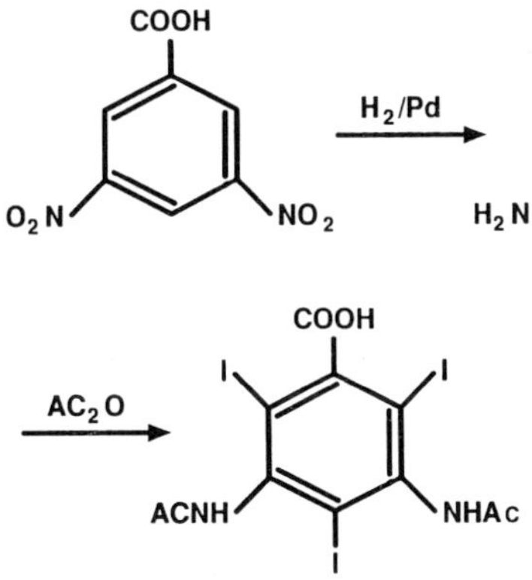

Fig. 1.2.2. Synthesis of diatrizoic acid
AC = Acetylation; Pd = Palladium Catalysis

Regarding nonionic media, as these are amide derivatives of the ionic media at least two more synthetic steps are needed to introduce the amide groups. Amidation may be accomplished at a late stage of the synthesis from the corresponding ionic compounds or, preferably, at an early stage before the iodine atoms are introduced (Fig. 1.2.3).

The price difference between nonionic and ionic CM reflects the cost of the two extra synthetic steps, along with the cost of hydroxylated amines.

Stereochemical Aspects of Contrast Media

Due to the large spatial requirements of the iodine atoms, rotations around the adjacent bonds to the aromatic ring is restricted (Fig. 1.2.4). For non-ionic CM in particular, this results in the existence of several stereoisomers

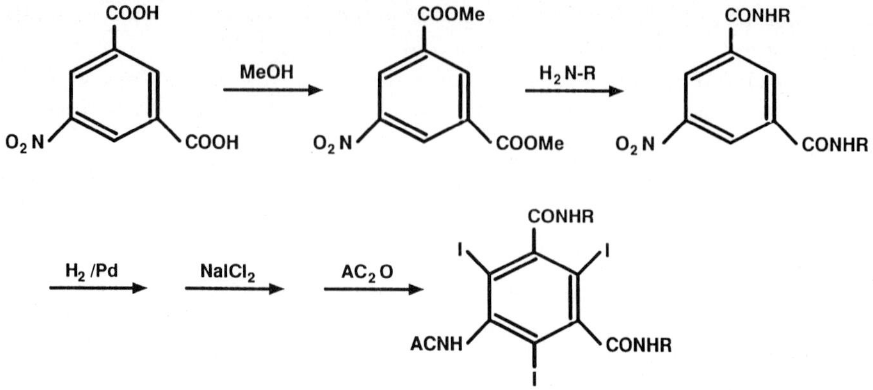

Fig. 1.2.3. Synthesis of nonionic contrast media. $R = CH_2CHOH\ CH_2OH$, Me = Methylation, Pd = Palladiun Catalysis

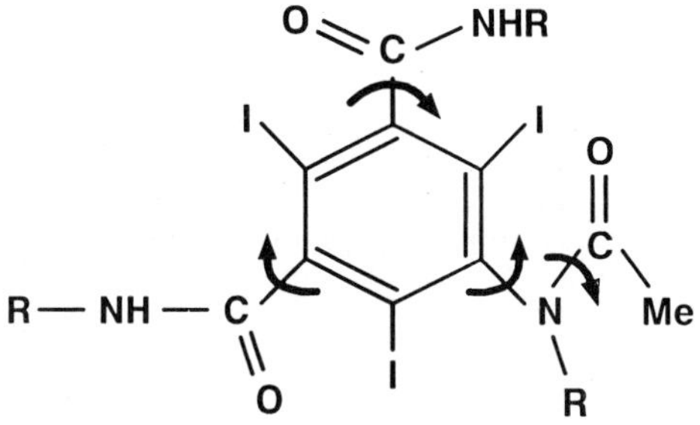

Fig. 1.2.4. Isomerism in iohexol. *Arrows* indicate hindered rotation. $R\ CH_2CHOHCH_2OH$

which can be separated by chromatographic techniques. A high number of stereoisomers contributes to the solubility of the compounds and for this reason nonionic CM have a higher solubility than could be predicted on the basis of the number of hydroxyl groups.

Oral Cholecystographic Agents

Oral cholecystographic agents must meet the following requirements:
– Absorption from the gastrointestinal tract
– Excretion into the bile at sufficient concentration
– Low toxicity, minimal adverse reactions

Figure 1.2.5 shows generalized structure of useful cholecystographic agents. They are normally triiodinated aromatics with one of the aromatic positions left unsubstituted and an aliphatic carboxylic group attached via a lipophilic link.

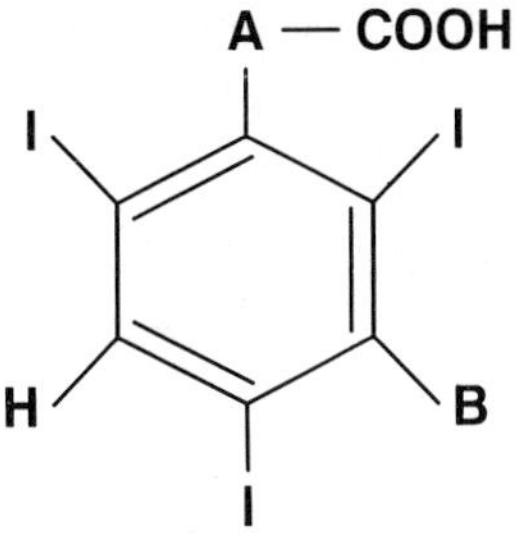

A — COOH

Fig. 1.2.5. Generalized structure of oral cholecystographic agents. A = lipophilic link, B = NH$_2$, NHAC etc.

References

1. Almén T (1989) Relations between chemical structure, animal toxicity and clinical adverse effects of contrast media. In: Enge I, Edgren J (eds) Patient safety and adverse events in contrast medium examinations. Elsevier/Excerpta Medica, Amsterdam (International Congress Series 816)
2. Sovak M (ed) (1984) Radiocontrast agents. Springer, Berlin Heidelberg New York (Handbook of Experimental Pharmacology vol 73)

1.3 Structure – Toxicity Relationships and Molecule Design

P. Dawson

There are two components to CM toxicity, one of which is well understood, namely high osmolality, and one of which is much less well understood, namely chemotoxicity. The former is a nonspecific effect which is a function only of the strength of the solution; the second is molecule – specific and depends on a number parameters of molecular structure.

It seems that CM exert their molecule-specific toxicity by way of weak nonspecific binding to biological macromolecules. This binding appears to be largely mediated through the hydrophobic portions of the molecule, the hydrophilic portions being solvated in water solution. The benzene ring – iodine core of the molecule is the principal hydrophobic portion. The extent to which this is available for interactions with biological molecules is variously measured as the partition coefficient (a measure of relative hydrophilicity/hydrophobicity), as protein binding capacity (e. g. with albumin) or, indirectly, as the magnitude of the effect on functional proteins, namely enzymes. A second and very important mechanisms of interaction between some contrast agents and biological macromolecules is the charge or Coulomb effect. This is not present, of course, with the nonionic agents which, by definition therefore, can be expected to be more inert, before any other considerations are taken into account.

Studies in this area have led to the conclusion that the design principles for a low-toxicity CM include the following:
1. The agent should be nonionic.
2. Hydrophilic substituents should be many and should mask the benzene ring – iodine core of the molecule.
3. The molecule should be compact so that the viscosity is not too high.
4. There should be isomerism in the molecule for reasons of entropy and solubility.

This subject is incomplelety understood but recent progress has been significant and the point may soon be reached where computer-aided design of molecules will be a realistic proposition.

1.4 Results of Toxicological Tests Assessing the Risk of Nonionic Contrast Media in Humans

C. Schöbel and *P. Günzel*

Introduction

In estimating the risk of new iodinated X-ray CM, animal experiments represent an important first step to be taken before clinical tests involving humans are started.

The programmes of toxicological tests performed for this purpose do not usually differ from those utilized to test any drug that is about to be released. Such a test programme for CM involves tests for the following:
– Acute toxicity
– Systemic tolerance during repeated administration
– Genotoxicity
– Reproductive toxicology
– Local tolerance
– Anaphylactoid reactions

We have already issued repeated reports on the character and performance of such studies [9–13, 31, 41, 42, 44–46]. For this reason, in the following, only representative findings from these types of studies (see list) performed to assess their risk in humans on the X-ray CM listed in Table 1.4.1.

Acute Toxicity Tests

Iodinated nonionic X-ray CM are usually characterized by a low level of acute toxicity. This can mainly be attributed to their metabolic stability, their quick and complete elimination and their low reactivity with biological

Table 1.4.1. Nonionic X-ray CM contrast media

Generic name	Trade name
Iohexol	Omnipaque
Iopamidol	Iopamiro(n) Solutrast
Iopromide	Ultravist
Metrizamide	Amipaque
Iotrolan	Isovist

systems. After intravenous administration, the LD_{50} values in dogs, rats and mice for all of the X-ray CM cited in Table 1.4.1 are > 10 g I/kg.

The absolute LD_{50} values of the various X-ray CM will not be cited here since as yet there is no comparative test of acute toxicity for all of the compounds listed (a test of all five X-ray CM in the course of one examination). The findings that are available, each originating at the time a given X-ray CM was developed and performed by different investigators, can sometimes diverge from one another quite considerably, depending on the method used (on the speed of administration in particular, if given intravenously), the animals used and the large periods of time between the different studies.

Systemic Tolerance During Repeated Administration

Tests of systemic tolerance are very important in estimating human risk. The site of repeated administration is determined according to the planned diagnostic use in humans (intravenous, subarachnoidal, etc.). Due to the very low systemic availability of iodinated X-ray CM after oral administration, systemic tolerance tests are usually superfluous for repeated oral administration of gastrographic agents. For this reason, only results from systemic tolerance tests of repeated intravenous or subarachnoidal administration will be reported upon here.

Intravenous Tests

With all of the above-mentioned X-ray CM, even if the largest doses tested (2.4–4 g I/kg) iodine/kg) were repeatedly administered to rats, dogs and/or monkeys (for 3–5 weeks), no clear organotoxic findings could be observed. With the medium and/or high doses of a few of the X-ray CM, minor and toxicologically irrelevant changes in chemical or hematological parameters occurred. Only after the highest tested doses of iopromide were given to rats (3.7 g I/kg) and monkeys (3.0 g I/kg), respectively, was vacuolation of hepatocytes observed.

All the X-ray CM referred to in Table 1.4.1, if repeatedly administered (3–5 weeks) at ca. 1.4–5 times the diagnostic dose induced a dose-dependent vacuolation of the proximal renal tubular epithelial cells. It makes no sense to provide a ranking of the five X-ray CM in terms of their potential to produce this effect, given the different experimental designs, different investigators and the large periods of time between the individual studies. These changes, which were also observed following ionic X-ray CM administration, did not lead to a reduction in renal function in the above studies. They proved to be reversible in additional studies performed on rats after repeated intravenous administration, the time needed for the changes to reverse depending upon the size of the selected dose and the frequency of administration.

The pathogenesis of vacuolation of the proximal renal tubular epithelial cells is not as yet clear. Two possibilities are conceivable:

1. Iodinated X-ray CM are excreted by glomeruli. When administered in very high doses, small amounts can also be excreted by tubules but the X-ray CM taken up from the blood by the tubular cells can only be re-excreted very slowly.
2. A small proportion of the X-ray CM that is exclusively excreted by glomeruli is reabsorbed by the proximal renal tubules.

Electronmicroscopic tests [4] with ioxaglic acid (7.5 g I/kg) and iotrolan (6 g I/kg) indicate that the extreme vacuolation of the proximal renal tubular epithelium cells does not lead to structural changes in cell organelles. This may also be taken to hold true for other iodinated X-ray CM that induce a vacuolation of the proximal renal tubular epithelium cells; this argument by analogy is permissible since all of the X-ray CM cited in Table 1.4.1 have practically the same excretion kinetics and all are metabolically stable.

Moreau et al. [35] have described changes in the context of water-soluble X-ray CM of vacuolation of the proximal renal tubular epithelium cells in renal biopsies of humans. They presume that these X-ray CM change the cellular metabolism in the kidney and this results in pinocytosis. Morphologically similar changes were observed in humans after intravenous administration of hyperosmolar sugar solutions and were termed "osmotic nephrosis". However, this term should not be used for iodinated X-ray CM, since such changes also occur in animal experiments using X-ray CM with lower osmolality or which are almost completely blood-isotonic.

The renal tolerance of X-ray CM is a special problem in their diagnostic use in humans [5, 29]. Reports mainly indicate temporary reduction in renal function, or rarely even renal failure. Presumably, these functional impairments can largely be attributed to local haemodynamic effects [43]. In animal experiments, even where there was extreme vacuolation of the proximal renal tubular epithelium cells, neither reduction of renal function nor indications of local haemodynamic effects were found. Thus, it doubtful that vacuolation of the proximal renal tubular epithelium cells has anything to do with the aforementioned changes in renal function.

On the basis of the findings from animal experiments, renal changes like vacuolation of the proximal renal tubular epithelium cells following administration of the usual one-off diagnostic dose in patients with normal renal function is not to be expected. Even if they do occur, they cannot be ascribed any disease-causing significance, since they have not been proven to induce either functional impairment or chronic changes; what has been shown clearly, is that their effects are reversible.

Subarachnoidal Tests

The nonionic X-ray CM listed in Table 1.4.1 do not usually pass the blood–brain barrier when the vascular endothelium is intact but the neural tolerance of those X-ray CM that are directly introduced into the CNS for such diagnostic purposes as myelography or ventriculography must be particularly thoroughly tested.

Separate animal studies with nonionic X-ray CM that have been developed for CNS studies are only available for iotrolan (300 mg I/ml), administered intracisternally (doses of 8, 40, 200 µl/animal each administered four times within 14 days to rats) and administered subarachnoidally in the lumbar region to dogs (doses of 0.13, 0.3, 0.83 mg/kg administered four times at 1-week intervals). In both species, no iotrolan-induced effects were observed, even after the highest tested dose was administered. In particular, there were no leptomeningeal changes (see also "Local Tolerance").

Genotoxicity and Reproductive Toxicology

No indications of reproductive or genotoxic effects have been found in risk assessment studies performed with the above-cited X-ray CM.

Local Tolerance

Human risk assessment tests were performed to determine the local tolerance of concentrations used diagnostically at the normal administration site and in tissue with which the X-ray CM might accidentally come into contact (as a result of misadministration, aspiration, perforation, and so on).

The good vascular tolerance (in arteries and veins) of all the compounds listed in Table 1.4.1 has been verified by means of clinical observation and histological testing of the administration sites in specially performed studies, such as local tolerance tests on rabbit ears (i. v., i. a.) and systemic tolerance tests with repeated administration (i. v.) to two, and in a few cases even three, species.

Specific comparative local tolerance tests were carried out on sensitive tissues, such as muscle and paravenous tissue (rabbit) and peritoneum (rat). The nonionic compounds iotrolan, iopamidol, iopromide and iohexol, each containing 300 mg I/ml, did not differ from one another in terms of the tissue tolerance found in paravenous and peritoneal tissue. Differences among the nonionic test preparations were confined to the very sensitive muscle tissue of the rabbit (see Table 1.4.2). Here iotrolan proved to be the best tolerated of the X-ray CM tested, there being practically no difference between it and the 0.9% (w/v) NaCl solution also tested.

It was only following paravenous administration that the ionic X-ray CM meglumine diatrizoate (Angiografin, 306 mg I/ml), which was included in each of these comparative tests, was clearly more poorly tolerated than the nonionic X-ray CM.

X-ray CM that are administered subarachnoidally in lumbosacral myelography can cause not only symptoms of acute irritation, but even symptoms of chronic meningeal intolerance, such as proliferation of granulation tissue. Such a proliferative change can then be imaged by means of repeated myelography, where it appears as obliterations of the nerve root sacs or as narrowing or shortening of the lumbar sac [1, 2, 14, 24, 27, 28, 32, 34]. The quantity of X-ray CM administered (longer retention time) and/or the osmotic behaviour of the cerebrospinal fluid (CSF) – X-ray CM mixture (dehydration of cells) might be the cause of these changes. No leptomen-

Table 1.4.2. Results of a comparative local tolerance test on a rabbit after the intramuscular administration of X-ray CM contrast media (eight administration sites/test solution; histological examinations of four administration sites on both days 3 and 7 after administration)

Designation (trade name)	Osmolality at 37°C (osmol/kg H_2O)	Degree of local irritation
0.9% (w/v) NaCl solution, isotonic salt solution (control)		Very marginal
Iotrolan (Isovist)	320	Very marginal to marginal
Iohexol (Omnipaque 300)	690	Marginal
Iopromide (Ultravist 300)	610	Marginal to medium
Iopamidol (Solutrast 300)	640	Medium
Meglumine diatrizoate (Angiografin)	1530	Medium

gineal changes were observed in humans after myelographies with metrizamide [2, 3, 6, 8, 14, 33, 48, 49]. Irstam [25] and Schmidt [47] claim that such changes are extremely rare; they have not yet been observed following iotrolan administration.

In experiments on monkeys, leptomeningeal changes after subarachnoidal introduction of the iodinated X-ray CM metrizamide, iopamidol and iohexol (nonionic) and of iocarmic acid (ionic, dimeric) into the lumbar regional were studied [15–23, 27]. Such changes occurred after metrizamide was administered ($\geq$ 1.2 ml; 300 mg I/ml), but even as the volume administered was increased with the same or higher iodine content, the changes were never more than moderate [19, 21], and they were always less marked than those induced by iocarmic acid, which was also tested in some of the trials. No differences in local tolerance were observed between metrizamide [19, 21] and iopamidol [19] or iohexol [21] when these were administered in the same volume (1.2 ml/monkey) and the same iodine concentration (300 mg/ml). When the volume (3.6 ml/monkey) and iodine content (370 mg/ml) were increased, metrizamide (marginal to medium changes) was somewhat more poorly tolerated than iohexol tested at the same time (marginal changes) [23]. Iopamidol and iohexol (300 mg I/ml, 3 ml/animal) did not induce any local changes when administered intracisternally to the leptomeninges of a dog [40].

Iotrolan did not induce any leptomengineal changes after single or repeated subarachnoidal administration of high volumes to the lumbar region (4 times at intervals of 1 week) in the dog (0.83 ml/kg = 10 ml/12 kg dog) or after repeated intracisternal administration to rats (doses of 8, 40, 200 µl/rat administered four times) [42].

For X-ray CM that are also designed for use in bronchography, local tolerance tests in the lungs are necessary for risk assessment. Such studies are also required for orally administered X-ray CM. Here the risk of accidental aspiration, especially in patients with dysphagia and in children, has to be assessed.

Comparative lung tolerance studies were performed on dogs with Isovist 300 (iotrolan), Ultravist 300 (iopromide), and Angiografin (meglumine diatrizoate; 306 mg I/ml) [39]. The animals each received one intrabronchial dose (0.6 ml/kg). Lung weights and oxygen partial pressure (PO_2) in the arterial blood were determined and histological analyses performed in order to assess lung tolerance. To this end, subgroups were sacrificed 2, 24 and 48 h after administration. The following ranking of tolerance was produced on the basis of these findings, with the best-tolerated X-ray CM listed first:

Ringer's solution $\geq$ Isovist 300 (iotrolan) > Ultravist 300 (iopromide) >> Angiografin (meglumine diatrizoate).

On the basis of these findings, it is recommended that iotrolan be developed as a bronchographic agent. For gastrointestinal studies with iodinated X-ray CM in problem patients with dysphagia iotrolan should be given preference.

Test for Detecting Anaphylactoid Reactions

Following the administration of iodinated X-ray CM, anaphylactoid reactions can occur in humans in the form of circulatory failure, nausea, vomiting, oedema, bronchoconstriction and so on. The mechanisms triggering such reactions are still not clear. Such reactions were not observed experimentally with any of the X-ray CM listed in Table 1.4.1, even with subchronic use (4 weeks), in the tested animal species (rats, dogs and monkeys).

Suitable animal models for detecting anaphylactoid reactions are to date still lacking; moreover, not only have the causal relationships in humans not been explained, they have not even been determined. As long as this holds, we are left with only one indication of the possible occurrence of such reactions; the examination of histamine release from mast cells and the determination of complement activation. Here, the nonionic X-ray CM appear to activate these two systems to a lesser extent than ionic compounds [7, 30, 36–38]. Since appropriate test models are lacking, however, the frequency and severity of such reactions can only be looked into in the course of clinical work on humans.

References

1. Ahlgren P (1973) Long term side effects after myelography with watersoluble contrast media: Conturex, Conray Meglumine 282 and Dimer-X. Neuroradiology 6:206–211
2. Ahlgren P (1975) Amipaque myelography. The side effects compared with Dimer X. Neuroradiology 9:197–202
3. Ahlgren P (1980) Early and late side effects of water-soluble contrast media for myelography and cisternography: a short review. Invest Radiol 15 (Suppl):S264–S266
4. Battenfeld R (1980) Licht- und elektronenmikroskopische Untersuchungen der osmotischen Nephrose nach Applikation eines Röntgenkontrastmittels. Inaugural Dissertation, Tierärztliche Hochschule Hannover
5. Cigarroa RG et al (1989) Dosing of contrast material to prevent contrast nephropathy in patients with renal disease. Am J Med 86:649–652
6. Chronqvist S (1977) Examination of the subarachnoid space with a water-soluble contrast medium (Amipaque). J Neuroradiol 4:13–27
7. Ennis M et al (1989) Histamine release from canine lung and liver mast cells induced by radiographic contrast media. Agents Actions 27:101–103
8. Graser C et al (1979) Zur Myelographie mit Metrizamid. Dtsch Med Wochenschr 104:511–514
9. Günzel P (1990) Schließen vom präklinischen Experiment auf den Menschen. In: Kuemmerle HP et al (eds) Klinische Pharmakologie, Bd 1, II-2.4.8, 4. Aufl, 24. Erg Lfg 2/90. Ecomed, Landsberg
10. Günzel P (1990) Grundsätzliche Überlegungen zur Durchführung experimenteller toxikologischer Untersuchungen. In: Kuemmerle HP et al (eds) Klinische Pharmakologie, Bd 1, II-2.4.1, 4. Aufl, 24. Erg Lfg 2/90. Ecomed, Landsberg
11. Günzel P, Schöbel C (1984) Systemische Verträglichkeitsprüfung bei einmaliger Verabreichung – akute Toxizitätsprüfung. In: Kuemmerle HP et al (eds) Klinische Pharmakologie, Bd 1, II-2.4.2, 4. Aufl. Ecomed, Landsberg
12. Günzel P et al (1986) Zur toxikologischen Prüfung von Kontrastmitteln. In: Burger OK et al (eds) Aktuelle Probleme der Biomedizin. Gruyter, Berlin, pp 275–288

13. Günzel P (1991) Diagnostika (Röntgen- u.a. Kontrastmittel). In: Hess R (eds) Arzneimitteltoxikologie, Anforderungen, Verfahren, Bedeutung. Thieme, Stuttgart, pp 397–404
14. Hansen EB et al (1978) Late meningeal effects of myelographic contrast media with special reference to metrizamide. Br J Radiol 51:321–327
15. Haughton VM et al (1977) Arachnoiditis following myelography with metrizamide in monkeys. Effect of blood in the cerebrospinal fluid. Acta Radiol Suppl 355:373–378
16. Hauhgton VM et al (1977) Experimental production of arachnoiditis with water-soluble myelographic media. Radiology 123:681–685
17. Haughton VM et al (1977) Arachnoiditis following myelography with water-soluble agents. Radiology 125:731–733
18. Haughton VM et al (1978) Comparison of arachnoiditis produced by meglumine locarmate and metrizamide myelography in an animal mdoel. Am J Roentgenol 131:129–132
19. Haughton VM, Ho KC (1980) The risk of arachnoiditis from experimental nonionic contrast media. Radiology 136:395–397
20. Haughton VM, Ho KC (1982) Arachnoid response to contrast media: a comparison of iophendylate and metrizamide in experimental animals. Radiology 143:699–702
21. Haughton VM et al (1982) Experimental study of arachnoiditis from iohexol, and investigational nonionic aqueous contrast medium. Am J Neuroradiol 3:375–377
22. Haughton VM, Ho KC (1982) Effect of blood on arachnoiditis from aqueous myelographic contrast media. Am J Roentgenol 139 (3):569–570
23. Haughton VM (1985) Intrathecal toxicity of iohexol vs. metrizamide. Survey and current state. Invest Radiol 20 (Suppl 1):S14–S17
24. Irstam L, Rosencrantz M (1974) Water-soluble contrast media and adhesive arachnoiditis. Acta Radiol 15:1–15
25. Irstam L (1978) Lumbar myelography with amipaque. Spine 3:70–82
26. Irstam L et al (1974) Lumbar myelography and adhesive arachnoiditis. Acta Radiol Diagn 15:356–368
27. Johansen JG et al (1984) Arachnoiditis from myelography and laminectomy in experimental animals. Am J Neuroradiol 5:97–99
28. Jorgensen J et al (1975) A clinical and radiological study of chronic lower spinal arachnoiditis. Neuroradiology 9:139–144
29. Kröpelin T et al (1983) The risk liability of nephrotropic contrast media: clinical and experimental results. In: Taenzer V, Zeitler E (eds) Contrast media in urography, angiography and computerized tomography. Thieme, Stuttgart, pp 129–142
30. Lang JH et al (1976) Activation of serum complement by contrast media. Invest Radiol 11:303–308
31. Lang R (1990) Prüfung auf genotoxische Wirkung. In: Kuemmerle HP et al (eds) Klinische Pharmakologie, Bd 1, II-2.4.5, 4. Aufl, 24. Erg Lfg 2/90. Ecomed, Landsberg
32. Liliequist B, Lundström B (1974) Lumbar myelography and arachnoiditis. Neuroradiology 7:91–94
33. McCormick CC et al (1981) Myelography with metrizamide. An analysis of the complications encountered in cervical, thoracic and lumbar myelography. Aust NZ J Med 11:645–650
34. McNeill TW et al (1976) A new advance in water-soluble myelography. Spine 1:72–84
35. Moreau JF et al (1980) Tubular nephrotoxicity of water-soluble iodinated contrast media. Invest Radiol 15 (Suppl 6):S54–S60
36. Muetzel W, Speck U (1983) Tolerance and biochemical pharmacology of iopromide. In: Taenzer V, Zeitler E (eds) Contrast media in Urography, Angiography and Computerized Tomography. Thieme, Stuttgart, New York, pp 11–17
37. Muetzel W, Speck U (1983) Tolerance and biochemical pharmacology of iopromide. Fortschr Geb Röntgenstr Nuklearmed 118:11–17
38. Muetzel W, Speck U (1983) Pharmacochemical profile of iopromide. Am J Neuroradiol 4:350–352

39. Müller N et al (1991) Results of a comparative pulmonary tolerance study in the dog following a single intrapulmonal application of three iodine-containing X-ray contrast media (Isovist-300, Ultravist-300, Angiografin). (in press)
40. Pasaouglu A et al (1988) An experimental evaluation of response to contrast media. Pantopaque, iopamidol, and iohexol in the subarachnoid space. Invest Radiol 23:762–766
41. Poggel HA (1984) Reproduktionstoxikologische Untersuchungen. In: Kuemmerle HP et al (eds) Klinische Pharmakologie, Bd 1, II-2.4.6, 4. Aufl. Ecomed, Landsberg
42. Press WR et al (1989) Tolerance to iotrolan after subarachnoid injection in animals. Fortschr Geb Röntgenstr Nuklearmed 128:126–133
43. Scherberich JE et al (1991) Unerwünschte Kontrastmittelwirkungen an der Niere. In: Peters PE, Zeitler E (eds) Röntgenkontrastmittel. Springer, Berlin Heidelberg New York, pp 65–69
44. Schöbel C, Günzel P (1984) Systemische Verträglichkeitsprüfungen bei wiederholter Verabreichung – subakute und chronische Toxizitätsprüfung. In: Kuemmerle HP et al (eds) Klinische Pharmakologie, Bd 1, II-2.4.3, 4. Aufl. Ecomed, Landsberg
45. Schöbel C, Siegmund F (1984) Lokale Verträglichkeitsprüfungen. In: Kuemmerle HP et al (eds) Klinische Pharmakologie, Bd 1, II-2.4.7, 4. Aufl. Ecomed, Landsberg
46. Schöbel, C, Günzel P (1991) Methoden und Ergebnisse toxikologischer Prüfungen von nichtionischen Röntgenkontrastmitteln. In: Peters PE, Zeitler E (eds) Röntgen-kontrastmittel. Springer, Berlin Heidelberg New York, pp 5–7
47. Schmidt RC (1980) Mental disorders after myelography with metrizamide and other water-soluble contrast media. Neuroradiology 19:153–157
48. Skalpe IO (1978) Adhesive arachnoiditis following lumbar myelography. Spine 3:61–64
49. Skalpe IO (1977) Lumbale Myelographie mit wasserlöslichen Kontrastmitteln (Metrizamid). Akt Neurol 4:179–183
50. Slätis P et al (1974) Hyperosmolality of the cerebrospinal fluid as a cause of adhesive arachnoiditis in lumbar myelography. Acta Radiol Diagn 15:619–629
51. Tirone P, Boldrini E (1983) Effects of radiographic contrast media on the serum complement system. Arch Toxicol (Suppl 6):37–41

1.5 Physicochemical Properties of Contrast Media: Osmotic Pressure, Viscosity, Solubility, Lipophilicity, Hydrophilicity, Electrical Charge

U. Speck

Introduction

The most important physicochemical features of water-soluble, iodinated CM are their solubility, the viscosity and osmotic pressure of their solutions, the lipophilic or hydrophilic qualities of the molecules carrying the iodine, and their electrical charge (Table 1.5.1). This section describes the practical significance of these features [8]:

Water Solubility

Very high water solubility is an absolute requirement for the production of highly concentrated CM of good X-ray CM density. Meglumine salts are

Table 1.5.1 The most important physicochemical features of water-soluble iodinated contrast media

Feature	Significance
Solubility	Maximum possible concentration; sometimes means dissolving crystals before use
Viscosity	Speed of injection, infusion. In selective angiography, very viscous solutions can disturb micro-circulation
Osmotic pressure	Pain in some angiographic indications, endothelial damage, arachnoiditis (?) in myelography, bradycardia in cardioangiography, hypervolaemia after administration of high doses, diuresis
Lipophilia, lack of hydrophilia	Frequent general reactions (nausea, vomiting, allergy-like reactions), especially in high doses and with rapid injection; protein binding, hindrance of glomerular filtration, tubular secretion and of biliary excretion; permeation through cell membranes, enteral absorption
Electrical charge	Improvement of solubility, increase in hydrophilicity, epileptogenicity

generally more soluble than sodium salts. The solubility of nonionic CM results, as in sugars or peptides, from hydrophilic groups such as -OH and -(ONH-. Some CM on the market may crystallize at low temperatures: To dissolve these crystals, they have to be warmed before use.

Viscosity

Viscosity is a measure of the fluidity of solutions. It is measured in millipascals (mPa) per second, which are identical to the older unit, the centipoise (cP). Viscosity increases greatly with rising concentration and with falling temperature (Fig. 1.5.1).

Low viscosity means above all that the CM in question can be quickly injected without too much effort or pressure. This is advantageous in urography, allowing high plasma levels and subsequent rapid excretion to be achieved [4]. In some angiographic techniques (narrow catheter lumen, high rates of flow), low viscosity is crucial. Moreover, low-viscosity CM mix more rapidly and homogeneously with the blood and, in selective arteriography, flow better through the smaller vessels and capillaries when undiluted or slightly diluted [5]. Preparations containing iopromide or iopamidol are suitable low-viscosity CM for angiography, CT and urography. The sodium salts of ionic CM should also be mentioned here, although not without strong reservations, since they are so poorly tolerated by patients.

In certain investigations, high viscosity can be advantageous, for example if one seeks to coat surfaces or prevent too rapid dilution. In angiography, more viscous CM can produce somewhat longer-lasting and thus better

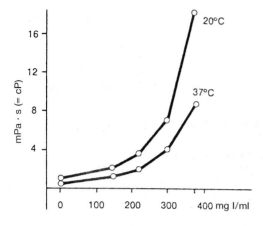

Fig. 1.5.1. Viscosity of Urografin (76%) as a function of concentration

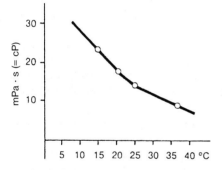

Fig. 1.5.2. Viscosity of Urografin (76%) as a function of temperature

contrast [7]. Since contact time with blood vessels is lengthened in this way, implementation of this principle presupposes very good local tolerance. CM with higher viscosity are the so-called dimers (hexaiodinated substances): these include, in addition to the intravenous biliary CM (e. g. iodipamide), the ionic compound sodium meglumine ioxaglate (Hexabrix) and the non-ionic CM iotrolan (Isovist) and iodixanol (Visipaque). At the same temperature and with the same iodine concentration, different CM have different viscosities (Figs. 1.5.1, 1.5.2).

Osmotic Pressure

The osmotic pressures of CM solutions are indicated in milliosmoles per kilogram of water, in megapascals or in atmospheres (1000 mOsm/kg = 2.58 MPa = 25.5 atm). The pressure is roughly proportional to the number of freely moving particles (molecules, ions) per kilogram water. The osmotic pressure of CM is strongly dependent upon the concentration and weakly

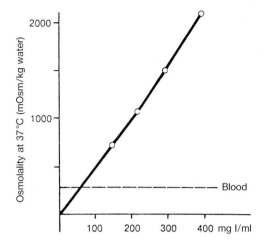

Fig. 1.5.3. Osmotic pressure as a function of concentration of Urografin 37 °C

dependent upon temperature (Fig. 1.5.3). Different CM with identical iodine concentrations can display very different osmotic pressures (Table 1.5.2). Most of the CM currently on the market are hypertonic compared to the blood at concentrations commonly used in angiography. Exceptions to this are diluted, so-called low-osmolar CM such as Ultravist 150 and Hexabrix 160 and, in particular, Isovist; the latter, even at 300 mg I/ml, is practically isotonic with blood and body fluids.

The high osmotic activity of standard ionic CM was one of the most important causes of side effects in vascular imaging when the solutions were not heavily diluted before use (phlebography and intraarterial digital subtraction angiography). In high intravenous doses and in body cavity imaging, many of the undesired effects can be ascribed to the high osmolality of most CM (Table 1.5.3) [1]. On the other hand, reactions such as nausea, vomiting, allergy-like reactions and certain cardiovascular effects are clearly not osmotically induced. They can also occur with highly diluted or even isotonic CM (such as cholegraphic media) or when very small amounts of CM are administered.

Lipophilicity

Lipophilicity refers to the affinity of molecules containing iodine for fats or lipid-dissolving agents and hydrophilicity to their affinity for water. The lipophilicity of CM acids containing iodine or of nonionic CM is determined by the way they distribute themselves between solvents non-miscible with water (Octanol, butanol) and an aqueous, buffer with a different pH value (distribution coefficient) (Fig. 1.5.4). By the 1950s, the connection between increasing tolerance and decreasing lipophilicity had been recognized [3]. At the same time, it was found that lipophilic CM (acids) tended to be

Table 1.5.2. Osmolality of ionic and nonionic contrast media at 37°C; mean ± 95% confidence interval)

Fluid	mg I/ml	Osmolality mOsm/kg water
Blood		290
Ionic CM		
Urografin 30%	146	710
45%	219	1050
60%	292	1500
76%	370	2100
Angiografin	306	1530
Urovist	306	1530
Ioxaglate	320	577 ± 13
(sodium meglumine)		
	160	ca. 300
	150	ca. 300
Nonionic CM		
Ultravist	240	483 ± 17
	300	607 ± 9
	370	774 ± 10
Iopamidol	200	437 ± 16
	300	607 ± 9
	370	774 ± 10
Omnipaque	240	525 ± 15
	300	685 ± 10
	350	823 ± 23
Amipaque	300	480

excreted by means of active transport processes, for example, biliary CM through the liver and the previously common urographic media through tubular excretion in the kidneys. Moreover, oral cholegraphic media have to be highly lipophilic in order to be enterally absorbed.

These features–toxicity and active transport–are obviously mediated by the increased binding to proteins in the body, including the transport proteins, that results from the lipophilicity of the molecules. The acid group of ionic CM plays a decisive role in this binding, even though their hydrophilicity is increased to a tremendous extent by it.

Nonionic X-ray CM are more lipophilic than comparable ionic urographic agents since they lack an acid group. They are, nevertheless, clearly better tolerated than the latter. Presumably, the low level of interaction between the neutral nonionic molecules and proteins, membranes and other biological substrates is more significant than lipophilic or hydrophilic factors.

Table 1.5.3. Pharmacological effects based on the hyperosmolality of CM

Angiography	Myelography
● Pain	● Depression/Sedation
● Damage to endothelium	● Pain
● Damage to blood-brain barrier	● Arachnoiditis
● Thrombosis and thrombophlebitis	
● Bradycardia and increase in contractility in angiocardiography	
● Increase in the pulmonary blood pressure	
● Vasodilatation and hypotension	

In any intravascular application of high CM doses	Other body cavities
● Vasodilatation and drop in blood pressure	● Fast dilution
● Hypervolemia	● Local inflammatory reactions
● Increase in diuresis	● Pulmonary edema
	● Increased peristalsis

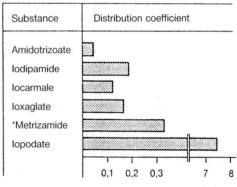

Fig. 1.5.4. Distribution coefficient of different X-ray CM between *n*-butanol (butanol) and a buffer (pH 7.6).

* Nonionic, only comparable to a limited extent

Electrical Charge

Ionic CM are salts of electrically negatively charged acids containing iodine. Positively charged cations do not contain any heavy elements; they thus do not contribute to the contrast density of the substances on the market, but can influence tolerance. Negatively charged CM acids and positively charged cations (e. g., Na^+ and $meglumine^+$) move independently of one another in the body and can also be excreted in different ways. The ionic character of the molecules influences their biological behaviour in a host of ways. In biliary CM, the use of the hepatic acid transport mechanism is, of course, premised upon it. In contrast, electrical charge is undesirable in CM used in angiography, urography and CT. It contributes to protein binding and the inhibition of enzymes. The calcium binding of CM acids increases the negative inotropic effect on the heart [6]. The better tolerance in many regards of nonionic CM has also been indisputably proven in the meantime in clinical tests [2]. Finally, the completely unsatisfactory tolerance of ionic CM in myelography should also be emphasized.

References

1. Grainger RG (1987) Osmolality and osmolality-related side effects. In: Contrast media from the past to the future. Berlin, March 27–28. Thieme, Stuttgart
2. Katayama H, Tanaka T (1988) Clinical survey of adverse reactions to contrast media. Invest Radiol 23:S88–S89
3. Knoefel PK, Huang KC (1956) The biochemorphology of renal tubular transport: iodinated benzoic acids. J Pharm Exp Ther 117:307–316
4. Mitchell DG, Friedman AC (1985) Viscosity of iodinated contrast agents: significance for peripheral venous injection. J Comput Tomogr 9:77–78
5. Morris TW, Kern MA, Katzberg RW (1982) The effects of media viscosity on hemodynamics in selective arteriography. Invest Radiol 17:70–76
6. Morris TW, Sahler LG, Fischer HW (1982) Calcium binding by radiopaque media. Invest Radiol 17:501–505
7. Nauert CM, Langer M, Mützel W (1989) Hemorrheologic effects of Iotrolan after intra-arterial injection in rabbits: comparison with other types of contrast media. Fortschr Geb Röntgenstrahl Nuklearmed Suppl 128:40–45
8. Speck U (1987) Newer perspectives in contrast media chemistry. In: Parvez Z, Moncada R, Sovak M (eds) Contrast media: biological effects and clinical application, vol 1. CRC Press, Boca Raton

1.6 Pharmacokinetics of Contrast Media

W. Krause and *G. Schuhmann-Gampieri*

Introduction

CM can be classified according to their contrast mechanism and the imaging technique with which they are to be used. For instance, iodinated CM are used for X-ray CM imaging, paramagnetic CM for MRI, radiopharmaceuticals for nuclear medicine and microbubbles for US. From a pharmacokinetic point of view, however, the pattern of biodistribution of CM is the most suitable form of classifications, distinguishing between extracellular fluid CM (ECF-CM; angiography, urography, myelography), hepatocellular or tissue-specific CM (e. g., cholangiography) and macromolecular CM that are confined to the vascular space (blood pool). At present, however, CM of this last type are not yet quite ready for release or are at an early research stage. Therefore blood pool enhancement has to be performed with extracellular fluid CM applying high doses and fast imaging techniques.

Table 1.6.1. Overview of contrast media (X-ray, MRI and nuclear medicine) with respect to their biodistribution

Extracellular fluid CM		Tissue-specific hepatobiliary CM	
Trade name	Generic name	Trade name	Generic name
Amipaque	Metrizamide	Bilimiro	Iopronic acid
Angiografin	Diatrizoate	Biliscopin	Iotroxic acid
Hexabrix	Ioxaglate	Biloptin	Iopodate
Imagopaque	Iopentol		
Isovist	Iotrolan	Cholebrine	Iocetamic acid
Magnevist	Gd-DTPA	Endomirabil	Iodoxamic acid
DOTAREM	Gd-DOTA		
Omnipaque	Iohexol	Telepaque	Iopanoic acid
Omniscan	Gadodiamide	–	Gd-EOB-DTPA
Optiray	Ioversol		
Prohance	Gadoteridol	–	Gadobenate
Iopamiron, Niopam	Iopamidol		dimeglumine
Ultravist	Iopromide	–	Mn-DPDP
Urografin	Diatrizoate		
Urovison	Diatrizoate		
Urovist	Diatrizoate		
–	^{51}Cr-EDTA		
–	^{99m}Tc-DTPA		

Abbreviations: Gd-DTPA, gadolinium diethylenetriaminepentaacetate (gadopentetate); EDTA, ethylenediaminetetraacetate; Gd-EOB-DTPA, Gd-ethoxybenzyl-DTPA; Mn-DPDP, manganese dipyridoxyldiphosphate

Extracellular Fluid Contrast Media

In general, ECF-CM are either negatively charged ionic molecules (Urografin, Angiografin, Urovist, Hexabrix for X-ray; Magnevist for MRI) or non-ionic molecules (Ultravist, Niopam, Omnipaque, Isovist, Amipaque for X-ray; Prohance, Omniscan for MRI, Table 1.6.1). Very high water solubility, low distribution coefficients between butanol and buffer and low binding to plasma proteins ($< 5\%$) are the main features of ECF-CM. After intravenous administration ECF-CM are rapidly distributed between the vascular and the interstitial spaces with a distribution half-life of about 3–10 min [11, 19, 20]. The ECF-CM are cleared from the blood with an elimination half-life of about 1.5–2 h [11, 19, 20]. The major organ of elimination is the kidney, glomerular filtration being the main process of renal elimination. The renal and total blood clearance are therefore close to the individual's creatinine clearance. Consequently, attempts have been made to use ECF-CM for assessment of renal function [4, 6]. In patients with normal renal function the extrarenal elimination of ECF-CM is low (< 2%).

Since ECF-CM are not distributed to any great extent into the intracellular compartment, the volume of distribution of an ECF-CM is about 0.25 l/kg, a value which typically represents the extracellular fluid space. No passage through the erythrocyte membrane occurs, and in man biotransformation has not been observed for any ECF-CM so far. Neither does measurable enterohepatic recirculation occur. In the dose ranges investigated, the pharmacokinetics were found to be linear or proportional to the dose [19].

In general, transfer of ECF-CM to human milk is low. Thus the daily dose a suckling infant would ingest is reported to be at most 0.05% of the administered dose for the ionic CM Angiografin and Magnevist, while for the nonionic CM Omnipaque a maximum of 0.5% was reported [3, 12]. Results from animal studies clearly indicate that passage through the placental barrier and through the intact blood – brain barrier can mostly be excluded for ECF-CM. After oral use, absorption of ECF-CM from the gastrointestinal mucosa is low and so diatrizoate could not only be developed for intravascular use (Urografin, Angigrafin) but also as a drinking solution (Gastrografin) to fill the bowel for imaging of the gastrointestinal tract.

Since glomerular filtration is the predominant route of elimination, the renal clearance of ECF-CM is reduced in renally impaired patients, thus increasing the elimination half-life. For Magnevist the renal clearance was reduced from 120 ml/min (normal renal function) to 20 ml/min or less, depending on the degree of renal failure and the patient's glomerular filtration rate (GFR) [8]. Consequently, the typical value of 1.5 h for the elimination half-life of an ECF-CM increased to 10 h or more, as is demonstrated in Figure 1.6.1 for both Magnevist and Iopamidol [5, 13]. Nevertheless, despite the increased residence time of the ECF-CM in the body of the renally impaired patient, elimination was prolonged but complete for both nonionic X-ray CM and Magnevist [5, 13] and renal tolerance was good. Only in patients with severely impaired renal function (GFR < 20 ml/min) might haemodialysis be necessary for shortening the elimination half-life and it has proved to be efficient and safe for many ECF-CM, e. g. Angiografin, Omnipaque, Ultravist and Magnevist [1, 7, 8, 18].

[51]Cr and ^{99m}Tc are often used as radionuclides in nuclear medicine. Intravenous administration of the free metal ions would result in uptake in the liver, spleen and bone, but complexing with the hydrophilic chelates diethylenetriaminepentaacetate (DTPA) and ethylenediaminetetraacetate (EDTA) changes the pharmacokinetics in the desired way. ^{99m}Tc-DTPA or ^{51}Cr-EDTA show very high water solubility, low protein binding, distribu-

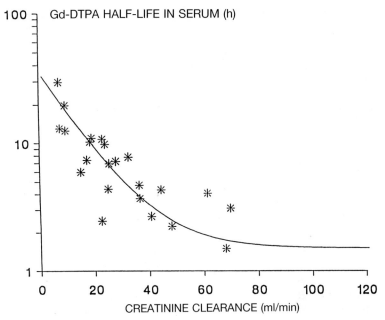

Fig. 1.6.1. Relation between creatinine clearance and elimination half-life of Magnevist (Gd-DTPA) in serum after single intravenous administration of 0.1 mmol/kg in patients with chronic renal failure. The fitted line approaches the elimination half-life of 1.5 h when renal function is normal (creatinine clearance of 120 ml/min). The same curve was observed when iopamidol (Niopam) was given to patients with chronic renal failure at a dose of 18 g I [9].

tion into the extracellular fluid space and rapid elimination from the body by glomerular filtration when administered intravenously. From a pharmacokinetic point of view these chelates are ECF-CM as well, and consequently the basic pharmacokinetic principles and features outlined above can be applied to [99m]TC-DTPA or ^{51}Cr-EDTA. The basic pharmacokinetic features of ECF-CM are summarized in Table 1.6.2.

Tissue-Specific Contrast Media

Hepatobiliary Contrast Media

Tissue specificity has been the goal for many therapeutic and diagnostic drugs. Targeting of the drug to the tissue of interest should reduce both the dose necessary to yield a certain drug concentration there and the side effects since no major distribution to and interaction with other tissues should occur. Interestingly, this goal has essentially been reached for the

Table 1.6.2. Summary of the pharmacokinetic features of extracellular fluid contract media

High hydrophilicity
Very low binding to plasma proteins ($< 5\%$)
Predominantly renal elimination through glomerular filtration
Elimination half-life of 1.5–2 h
Very little extrarenal elimination ($< 2\%$)
Pharmacokinetics linear or proportional to dose
No biotransformation
No enterohepatic circulation
Prolonged but complete elimination in renal insufficiency
Dialysable
Negligible passage of the blood–brain and placental barrier
Little enteral absorption

iodinated hepatobiliary CM: apart from being distributed into the extracellular fluid space, these agents are only distributed intracellularly in the hepatocytes. Although they are useful for cholecystography and cholangiography, the concentration achieved in the hepatocytes is not sufficient to provide useful contrast enhancement in the liver. In general, iodinated hepatobiliary CM are negatively charged ionic molecules that are less hydrophilic than ECF-CM due to an appropriate chemical substitution [2]. This balance between hydrophilic and lipophilic features allows the iodinated hepatobiliary CM to dissolve in the intestinal lumen, be absorbed and distributed into the extracellular fluid space and be taken up by the hepatocytes and excreted via the bile. The monomeric hepatobiliary CM are designed for oral use (Biloptin, Cholebrine, Bilimiro, Telepaque; Table 1.6.1) whereas the dimeric hepatobiliary CM are for intravenous use (Biliscopin, Endomirabil; Table 1.6.1).

In general, the solubility in water of the oral iodinated hepatobiliary CM at physiological pH values is low, ranging from 0.6 mmol/l to about 30 mmol/l (the water solubility of ECF-CM is in the order of 500 to 1000 nmol/l). As a consequence of the lower hydrophilicity, iodinated hepatobiliary CM exhibit considerable plasma protein binding, which at the same time, however, seems to be important in increasing the solubility in plasma and prevents premature renal excretion. Plasma binding of iodinated hepatobiliary CM is of the order of 70%–95% and appears to be saturable (nonlinear) since binding clearly depends on the CM concentration [15, 16].

Administered intravenously, iodinated hepatobiliary CM are reversibly and nonspecifically bound to plasma proteins, and an equilibrium is established between the free, unbound CM concentration and the bound CM concentration in the blood. The free, unbound CM is better able to leave the intravascular space, is freely distributed into the interstitial space and at the same time undergoes glomerular filtration via the kidneys. Of the total dose of iodinated hepatobiliary CM administered, 10%–35% is excreted renally [15]. Besides being eliminated renally – a process which for most iodinated hepatobiliary CM has been shown to be linear or nonsaturable [2] – the majority of the free unbound CM is specifically taken up by the hepatocytes and excreted into the bile, which makes the CM suitable for cholangiography. This process of biliary excretion, however, proved to be saturable for all iodinated hepatobiliary CM in the diagnostic dose range applied. Saturation or inhibition of biliary excretion was reported from intensive studies using increasing doses or coadministering compounds competing for the same transport mechanism across the hepatocyte membrane, e.g. sulphobromophthalein bilirubin or even other hepatobiliary CM [10].

Extrarenal elimination due to biliary excretion plays a major role in the disposition of the iodinated hepatobiliary CM in the body. The liver can clear the blood of compounds in a single pass. This phenomenom is called a "first-pass effect": it occurs especially with the orally administered iodinated hepatobiliary CM since a substantial proportion of the dose is cleared by the liver before the CM reaches the systemic circulation. However, it must be taken into consideration that for a drug with high hepatic clearance this parameter, and consequently the plasma concentration, is heavily dependent on the liver blood flow of the individual. Because of this and because of interindividual variations in plasma protein binding, greater variability is observed in the pharmacokinetics of the iodinated hepatobiliary CM than with ECF-CM.

Iodinated hepatobiliary CM for oral use are less water soluble than the corresponding intravenous compounds and so appear to be more subject to biotransformation than the intravenously administered cholegraphic agents. iopodate (Biloptin) undergoes glucuronidation in the liver and is excreted via the bile as the more water soluble glucuronide species [2]. The glucuronidation also prevents reabsorption from the intestinal lumen (enterohepatic recirculation). Probably due to their higher lipophilicity, iodinated hepatobiliary CM are able to pass into human milk to a slightly greater extent than ECF-CM. For iopanoic acid the maximum amount an infant would ingest is reported to be 6.9% of the dose. Exposure of the infant may be limited by delaying breastfeeding for 24 h [3].

For MRI too, tissue-specific hepatobiliary contrast agents (lipophilic derivatives of the hyrophilic paramagnetic chelates) are under development and are presently being tested in clinical trials phase I–III. The three most advanced hepatobiliary CM for MRI are gadolinium-ethoxybenzyl-diethylenetriaminepentaacetate (Gd-EOB-DTPA), gadobenate dimeglumine, and manganese dipyridoxyldiphosphate (Mn-DPDP) [9, 14, 17]. Two basic differences make the hepatobiliary MRI CM better than the iodinated hepatobiliary CM discussed above: first, higher sensitivity of MRI means that the CM concentration necessary to obtain an increase in signal intensity in the liver is ten-fold lower, thus decreasing the diagnostic tissue concentration significantly; secondly, hepatobiliary MR CM are only slightly bound to plasma (about 10%) and there is no saturation in plasma binding within the

Table 1.6.3. Summary of the pharmacokinetic properties of hepatocellular contrast media

	X-ray	MRI
Hydrophilicity	Moderate	High
Plasma binding	High (70%–95%, saturable)	Low (10%)
Renal elimination	Low (10%–35%)	Moderate to high
Extrarenal (biliary) elimination	High	Low to moderate
Saturability of biliary excretion	Yes	Yes
Dose-dependent pharmacokinetics	Yes	Yes
Biotransformation	Partially observed	No
Enterophepatic recirculation	Partially observed	No

clinically useful range of doses and concentrations. This results in less variability in the pharmacokinetics between individual patients. The basic pharmacokinetic features of hepatobiliary CM are summarized in Table 1.6.3.

Contrast Media for the Reticuloendothelial System

CM for the reticuloendothelial system (RES CM) are not commercially available yet. However, many attempts have been made to direct particulate CM selectively to the Kupffer cells of the liver and spleen, basically in order to avoid distribution of the CM into the extracellular fluid space and thus decrease the dose needed for sufficient enhancement of liver and spleen. Three major approaches (Table 1.6.4) have been undertaken to obtain RES CM particles: first, encapsulation of the CM (Gd-DTPA as well as iopromide or diatrizoate) into liposomes; secondly, the synthesis of iron oxide particles (magnetites) for MRI; and third, making gas-containing microcapsules for ultrasound (US). From a pharmacokinetic standpoint, targeting of CM to the reticuloendothelial system raises many questions: Are there species differences in the relative weight of the liver and/or in the phagocytic activity? How does the particle size influence biodistribution? What is the effect of particle surface charge? Does saturation of uptake in the reticuloendothelial system occur or, in other words, are the pharmacokinetics of

Table 1.6.4. Characteristic of particulate contrast media for liver imaging

Modality Type of particle	X-ray MRI Liposomes	MRI Magnetites	US Microcapsules
Preparation	Entrapment of iodinated CM/Gd chelate	Superparamagnetic particles (Fe_3O_4) with hydrophilic coating	Stabilized air bubbles (polymer coating)
Target Tissue	RES	RES	RES
Elimination			
CM	Renal excretion	Biodegradation	Dissolution
Coating	Biodegradation	Biodegradation	Biodegradation

RES CM nonlinear and dose dependent? As yet only limited information is available to answer these questions and a lot of work remains to be done before we can understand and interpret the pharmacokinetic behaviour of RES CM better.

References

1. Ackrill P, McIntosh S, Nimmon C et al (1976) A comparison of the clearance of urographic contrast medium sodium diatrizoate by peritoneal and haemodialysis. Clin Sci Med 50:69–74
2. Barnhart JL (1984) Hepatic disposition and elimination of biliary contrast media. In: Sovak M (ed) Radiocontrast agents. Springer, Berlin Heidelberg New York, pp 367–418
3. Bennett PN, Bath FRCP (1988) Drugs and human lactation. Elsevier, Amsterdam
4. Choyke PL, Austin AH, Frank JA et al (1992) Hydrated clearance of gadolinium-DTPA as a measurement of glomerular filtration rate. Kidney Int 41:1595–1598
5. Corradi A, Menta R, Cambi V et al (1990) Pharmacokinetics of iopamidol in adults with renal failure. Arzneimittelforschung/Drug Res 40 (II):830–832
6. Effersoe H, Rosenkilde R, Groth S et al (1990) Measurement of renal function with iohexol or a comparison of iohexol, ^{99m}Tc-DTPA, and ^{51}Cr-EDTA clearance. Invest Radiol 25:778–782
7. Kierdorf H, Kindler J, Winterscheid R et al (1989) Elimination of the nonionic contrast medium iopromide in end-stage renal failure by haemodialysis. In: Taenzer V, Wende S (eds) Recent developments in nonionic contrast media. Thieme, Stuttgart New York, pp 119–123
8. Lackner K, Krahe T, Götz R, Haustein J (1990) The dialysability of gadolinium-DTPA. In: Bydder G, Felix R, Büchler E et al (eds) Contrast media in MRI. Medicom Europe, Bussum, pp 321–326
9. Lim KL, Stark DD, Leese PT et al (1991) Hepatobiliary MR imaging: first human experience with MnDPDP. Radiology 178:79–82
10. Lin KS, Moss AA, Riegelmann S (1979) Kinetics of drug-drug interactions: biliary excretion of iodoxamic acid and iopanoic acid in rhesus monkeys. J Pharm Sci 68:1430–1433
11. Mützel W, Nagel R, Kemper JD, Clauß W (1984) Pharmakokinetik des nichtionischen Röntgenkontrastmittels Iohexol. Akt Urol 15:154–156
12. Schmiedl U, Maravilla KR, Gerlach R, Dowling CA (1990) Excretion of gadopentetate dimeglumine in human breast milk. AJR 154:1305–1306
13. Schuhmann-Giampieri G, Krestin G (1991) Pharmacokinetics of Gd-DTPA in patients with chronic renal failure. Invest Radiol 26:975–979
14. Schuhmann-Giampieri G, Schmitt-Willich H, Press WR et al (1992) Preclinical evaluation of Gd-EOB-DTPA as a contrast agent in MR imaging of the hepatobiliary system. Radiology 183:59–64
15. Speck U, Mützel W, Herz-Hübner U, Siefert HM (1978) Pharmakologie der Iotroxinsäure eines neuen intravenösen Cholegraphikums. Arzneimittelforschung/Drug Res 28 (II):2143–2149
16. Taenzer V, Speck U, Wolf R (1977) Pharmakokinetik und Plasmaeiweißbindung von Iotroxinsäure. Fortschr Röntgenstr 126:262–267
17. Vogl TJ, Pegios W, McMahon C et al (1992) Gadobenate dimeglumine – a new contrast agent for MR imaging: preliminary evaluation in healthy volunteers. AJR 158:887–892
18. Waaler A, Svaland M, Fauchald P et al (1990) Elimination of iohexol, a low osmolar nonionic contrast medium, by hemodialysis in patients with chronic renal failure. Nephron 56:81–85

19. Weinmann HJ, Laniado M, Mützel W (1984) Pharmacokinetics of Gd-DTPA/dimeg-lumine after intravenous injection into healthy volunteers. Physiol Chem Phys Med NMR 16:167–172
20. Wolf KJ, Steidle B, Skutta T, Mützel W (1983) Iopromide. Clinical experience with a new non-ionic contrast medium. Acta Radiol 24:55–62

1.7 Clinical Documentation of the Tolerance, Safety and Efficacy of X-Ray Contrast Media

E. Andrew, W. Clauß, A. Alhassan, and H. P. Bohn

Prior to release for clinical use a new CM, must undergo a comprehensive preclinical in vitro and in vivo tests. Although LD_{50} assessments of CM in animals seem in contrast to therapeutic drugs in general, to correlate well with the tolerance experienced in patients, it is clinical experience [1] that really counts when the CM finally reaches human trials and clinical use.

The diagnostic use of CM is based on the physical ability of iodine to absorb X-ray, not on pharmacological effects, and is similar for all vascular CM based on iodinated chemical structures. Clinical trials with CM have therefore concentrated on the recording of adverse reactions and assessment of safety. However, diagnostic efficacy has also to be confirmed clinically.

Since clinical trials, and particularly randomized double-blind trials, are the accepted scientific method for evaluating safety and efficacy in man, the results serve as the basis for important decisions on CM by pharmaceutical companies, regulatory authorities and physicians.

New CM undergoing clinical testing have to pass through a very strict and meticulous clinical programme with step-wise advancement for safety reasons. Human beings with increasing range of disease are gradually included as the clinical trial programme progresses. For new CM, as for other drugs, the clinical trials up to marketing authorization are generally divided into three phases (Table 1.7.1). Each phase has to answer specially defined questions and so they are, in general, conducted sequentially, although they may overlap.

For the whole clinical trial programme up to submission of an NDA (New Drug Application) a time of 3–5 years is usually needed, although compared to long-term therapeutic drugs the clinical documentation of vascular CM is relatively uncomplicated.

The size of the patient population that a CM needs to be tested on to achieve release or market approval depends on the claims, the indications included and the regulatory authority involved. Usually, the number of the patients given the new CM varies roughly between 500 and 2000 patients in the first registration file. Additional indications documented later on may require fewer patients, depending on the claim. In Europe, documen-

Table 1.7.1 Clinical testing of contrast media

Clinical phase	Classification/definition	Aim
I	Initial introduction of a new CM into humans. The CM is given to a small number of preferably healthy male volunteers.	To gain a preliminary elucidation of the human pharmacological properties (pharmacokinetics, tolerance) before advance to diseased subjects.
II	Noncomparative, later possibly comparative, trials in the first small number of patients.	To determine the intended effect of the CM for a certain indication by approximating the doses used for the other CM to assess patient safety and tolerance.
III	Expanded, usually comparative, trials in larger (and possibly varied) patient group for the same indication as in phase II.	To gain additional and preferably comparative documentation about the efficacy and safety and, to evaluate the overall benefit–risk relationship.

tation of relative tolerability/safety and efficacy is usually required for registration purposes.

As a matter of principle, every clinical trial has to fulfil the ethical recommendations of the current version of the Declaration of Helsinki (World Medical Association Declaration of Helsinki in 1976). In addition, the health authorities of most countries have published regulations and/or guidelines.

The guidelines of the European Community (EC) of Good Clinical Practice (GCP) should raise the quality of European clinical trial documentation to the same level as in the USA. This will mean in practice that all procedures and the data produced must be verified and documented in detail to ensure the reliability of the data and to protect the subjects/patients involved. Contrary to the American Food and Drug Administration (FDA) guidelines and practices, the European GCP guidelines are to be applied for all trials (phases I–IV), not only preregistration trials. According to the GCP all trials must be approved by an ethical committee and in most European countries, the regulatory authorities will also assess the protocol before the trial starts. Nordic countries have similar guidelines for good clinical trial practice.

After marketing of the drugs the documentation process will continue in order to evaluate their usefulness in clinical practice and further assess the relative safety and effectiveness and cost – benefit ratio (phase IV clinical trials and postmarketing surveillance or PMS).

The possible injuries caused by a medical product are studied with a view to discovering the seriousness, outcome, frequency of occurrence, risk factors, drug–drug interactions, optimal treatment, dose relationship and long-term effects, the costs of these to society and to using this pharmaco-epidemiological information to minimize the risk of such injuries and in risk–benefit assessments.

All methods for monitoring the safety and efficacy of *marketed* drugs are included under PMS. They may be classified as follows:

A Nonanalytical, descriptive methods

1. Voluntary or mandatory spontaneous reporting
2. Uncontrolled studies

B Analytical methods

1. Experimental (clinical and toxicological)
2. Nonexperimental (epidemiological)
   a) Cohort survey (prospective or retrospective)
   b) Case-control study (prospective or retrospective)
   c) Disease trend study

C Literature surveillance

The spontaneous reporting system is the method generally used and the medical legislation of many countries makes this system obligatory. Doctors are requested to report events and adverse reactions occurring after the use of drugs. Special adverse drug reaction forms are used and are generally sent to the responsible pharmaceutical company. However, in some cases and in some countries the reports are sent directly to the drug regulatory authorities or to other agencies set up for monitoring such adverse events or reactions.

The pharmaceutical companies in most countries are obliged to forward such reports, either periodically or without delay, depending on the type of reaction and country, to the responsible health authority. Safety updates for the renewal of a marketing licence are also often requested from the pharmaceutical companies.

Under this system it is possible to monitor adverse events and reactions and suspected adverse reactions connected with the administration of a given drug. This contributes to the creation of a broader adverse reaction profile and updating of package inserts or data sheets, since the clinical trials usually detect only the more common adverse reactions. It also facilitates a risk–benefit assessment. Major disadvantages worth mentioning are that it does not enable the assessment of causality and it is extremely sensitive to bias, e. g. due to adverse publicity.

The other methods listed are generally employed when further clarification of questions arising from the spontaneous adverse event or reaction monitoring is necessary.

Interestingly, the incidence of CM adverse reactions in preregistration trials is 2–10 times higher than that recorded in PMS. The pattern of reaction is the same, so the difference probably reflects the greater scrutiny and vigilance in early clinical phases [2] compared with daily clinical routine.

The new modern CM such as nonionic media have a very low incidence of adverse effects, particularly of severe reactions. Accordingly, in order to establish a safety profile based on more medically important reactions, patient populations larger than those surveyed in preregistration trials are needed. The drug monitoring performed by Schrott et al. in Germany on 50,000 patients [3] and the surveys performed by Katayama et al. in Japan on 338,000 patients [4] and Palmer in Australia on 110,000 [5] patients have not only documented the superiority of nonionic over ionic CM in the incidence of the usual mild and moderate adverse effects found in pre-registration trials, but have also convincingly demonstrated that there are fewer medically serious reactions.

References

1. Andrew E (1989) Clinical relevance of toxicological experiments on drugs (in Norwegian, English summary). Nor Lægeforening 106:1935–1938)
2. Andrew E (1990) Adverse reactions of x-ray contrast media in pre-registration trials versus post-marketing surveillance (PMS). 2nd international symposium of CM, Osaka, Japan, November 1990
3. Good clinical practice for trials on medicinal products in the European Community. COMEUR, Brussels, 1990
4. Katayama H, Yamaguchi K, Kozuka T et al (1990) Adverse reactions to ionic and non-ionic contrast media. A report from the Japanese Committee on the Safety of Contrast Media. Radiology 11:52–66
5. Palmer FJ (1989) The Royal Australian College of Radiologists (RACR) survey of reactions to intravenous ionic and non-ionic media. In: Enge I, Edgren J (eds) Patient safety and adverse events in contrast medium examination. Elsevier, Amsterdam, pp 137–141 (Excerpta medica international Congress series, vol 816)
6. Schmitt KM, Behrends B, Clauß W, Kaufmann J, Lehnert J (1986) Iohexol in der Ausscheidungsurographie. Ergebnisse des Drug-monitoring. Fortschr Med 7:153–156

CHAPTER 2

Pharmaceutical Quality and Stability of Contrast Media

2.1 What Are the Steps in the Production of Contrast Media?

B. Wolden

The production process for sterile solutions of CM, which are often injected or infused in large volumes, can be thought of in terms of the following steps:
1. Preparation of the solution
2. Filtration
3. Filling
4. Sterilization
5. Visual inspection

Preparing the solution involves dissolving all ingredients (active substance and excipients) in water for injection. The pH is adjusted to approximately 7.

The solution is then *filtered* to remove: (a) visible particles; (b) invisible particles, which contribute to the overall particulate burden of the solutions and (c) particles as small as 0.2 μm, which include the bioburden of fungi and bacteria.

The solution is *filled* into washed vials or bottles that are closed with washed rubber stoppers and sealed. The vials or bottles are then *sterilized* at 121 °C for 15 min (autoclaving) and subsequently *inspected* for visible particulate matter.

2.2 Which Chemical Degradation Products Are Formed?

D. Herrmann

All X-ray CM that are based on triiodinated aromatic ring systems are capable of releasing iodide ions. Decomposition speed depends on the molecular structure of the CM compound and the composition of the X-ray CM solution (especially on its pH value), as well as on the temperature and light to which it is exposed. Elemental iodine is normally not released. The frequently observed yellowing of CM solutions is usually due to organic impurities or compounds that form as a result of overexposure to light or heat, and not to free iodine. The release of colourless iodide ions occurs in both ionic and nonionic CM, in sodium and meglumine salts of amidotrizoic acid or ioglycamic acid just as much as in nonionic compounds like iohexol, iopromide and iopamidol. The release of iodide is catalysed by heavy metal ions, which bind to the stabilizer calcium disodium edetate to form a complex. Figure 2.2.1 shows how iodide is released from amidotrizoic acid.

A further degradation reaction is the formation of primary aromatic

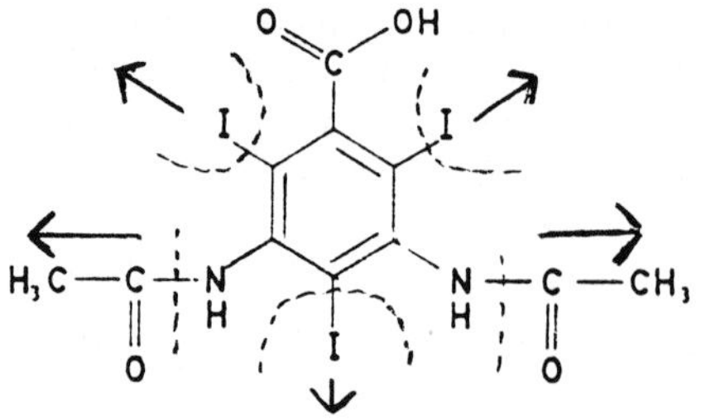

Fig. 2.2.1. Release of iodide and formation of an aromatic amine from amidotrizoic acid

amine compounds as a result of saponification of the amido bond. This reaction can of course only occur in CM compounds that have a primary amido group attached to an aromatic carbonic acid. Here, too, the reaction rate depends on the pH of the CM solution and the temperature; in contrast to iodide release, however, exposure to light has practically no influence.

Drops in pH are often observed in CM solutions following degradation reactions, i. e., a secondary reaction is involved. These drops in pH can then trigger further changes, for example the separation of CM acid from ionic CM solutions as a result of its being displaced from its salt bond by the stronger acids formed in the process of degradation.

2.3 What Additives Do Contrast Media Formulations Contain?

B. Wolden

For ready-made CM, and for parenteral products in general, any additive must be justified by a clear purpose and function. Buffers, chelating agents and electrolytes are included as additives in ready-made CM.

Buffers

The buffers that may be found in ready-made CM include citrates, phosphates and trometamol (TRIS). Buffers are included in some CM solutions to maintain a certain pH range in the solution when this is required to maintain stability of the active substance. The buffer capacity, however, of a parenteral product must be readily overcome by the biological fluids; thus, the concentration and ratios of buffers must be carefully selected.

Chelating Agents

Chelating agents that may be found in ready-made CM include ethylenediaminetetraacetic acid (edetate or EDTA) agents and salts of these, as well as citric acid. Chelating agents are added to complex, and thereby inactivate, metals such as copper, iron and zinc, which generally catalyse degradation (deiodination) of the active X-ray contrast substance. Possible sources of metal contamination include raw material impurities, solvents such as water, the packaging system, rubber stoppers or containers and equipment employed in the manufacturing process.

Electrolytes

Ionic CM, because of their ionic nature, contain ions or electrolytes in solution such as Na^+, Ca^{2+}, K^+ or Mg^{2+}. These electrolytes are said to have a positive effect on the tolerance of the ionic CM.

For nonionic CM, small amounts of electrolytes like Na^+, Ca^{2+}, K^+ or Mg^{2+} may be added in order to increase the tolerability of the preparation, but not of course in such a way as to greatly affect the osmolality of the solution, which should be close to isotonic.

2.4 What Is the Importance of Additives in Contrast Medium Formulations?

P. Dawson

Some of the conventional CM contain sodium citrate or sodium edetate. Both these materials are capable of binding calcium and undoubtedly play a role in the various manifestations of cardiotoxicity seen with these agents. Indeed, the addition of a little calcium to the formulation may largely eliminate the cardiotoxic effects in these compounds. It is important to note, also, that the anion in the ionic CM is itself also capable of binding calcium without the presence of additives.

The nonionic solutions contain no citrate and a different preparation of EDTA, namely calcium disodium edetate. Neither this additive nor the nonionic molecule itself is capable of significant calcium binding, and this undoubtedly is an important element in their significantly lower cardiotoxicity.

Recently, animal experiments have been performed which indicate that the absence of sodium ions in the nonionic CM formulations may lead to an increased incidence of ventricular fibrillation. It is important to understand that this appears only to be the case in experimental situations, which do not reflect at all well clinical practice in real coronary angiography. Indeed, after widespread use for some years in clinical coronary angiography worldwide, there has been no impression of any increase in ventricular fibrillation. However, these animal experiments have led to suggestions that sodium ions should be added to nonionic formulations in some way and some commercial companies are at least experimenting with the idea. The addition of sodium in the form of sodium chloride is one simple possibility. An alternative would be the addition of sodium citrate. This would not only supply the sodium ions deemed necessary to minimize the incidence of ventricular fibrillation but would also restore a calcium binding potential to the formulations. In so far as this would restore the strong anticoagulant effects which are routinely found in the ionic agents, but have been largely lost in the nonionic agents, this is thought by some authorities to be desirable. However, there appear to be at least two problems. First, the calcium binding not only mediates an anticoagulant effect but also, as indicated above, is largely responsible for cardiotoxicity. Such formulations might therefore be expected to be more cardiotoxic as regards effects on pump function and various aspects of electrophysiology, notwithstanding the original aim of reducing the incidence of ventricular fibrillation! The second problem is that the addition of significant amounts of sodium citrate in our laboratory studies appeared to markedly raise the osmolality of the solutions.

In short, the philosophy in the development of the nonionics has been to try to attain something close to the ideal of total inertness of CM formulations, and the addition of more active additives, or new additives, to achieve doubtful ends, while at the same time risking loss of the very inertness desired, seems a rather undesirable course on which to embark.

filtration chamber at 30°–35°C in order to detect bacteria and one filtration chamber at 20°–25°C in order to detect fungi. No growth of micro-organisms occurs if the product is sterile.

2. *Culture tube method:* CM is inoculated directly into a tube with culture medium, whose suitability for growth of micro-organisms and fungi has been shown. Incubation is as described in 1.

The membrane filter method is used for CM that show bacteriostatic properties, so as to permit separation of possible contaminating micro-organisms from growth inhibitors.

2.5 How Is the Sterility or Microbial Purity of Contrast Media Checked?

B. Wolden

The sterility of a CM production (a lot or batch) is checked by setting up a sterility test to determine the probable sterility. The testing can be performed by two different methods:

1. *Membrane filter method:* CM is filtered through two membrane filtration chambers having a pore size not greater than 0.45 µm, whose effectiveness to retain micro-organisms have been established. The membranes are rinsed to remove residues, and two culture media are sequentially introduced into the filtration chambers. The filtration chambers are incubated for not less than 7 days, one

2.6 How Is the Chemical Stability of Contrast Media Checked?

B. Wolden

Decomposition, e. g. deiodination, of ready-made CM can be detected on the basis of changes in iodide ion concentrations, pH and the colour of the solution [1]. The chemical stability of the CM is checked by monitoring these changes via different analytical methods (Table 2.6.1). The monitoring is performed as release controls on each batch of CM produced, and as follow-up controls on a number of batches stored under conditions of time and temperature relevant for practical use.

Table 2.6.1. Analytical methods used for monitoring chemical stability of contrast media

Parameter change	Analytical method
Iodide ion	Titration with silver nitrate
pH	pH measured directly in solution at a definite temperature
Colour change	Absorbance against purified water in UV/visible spectroscopy
Quantity of active substance	HPLC (High Performance Liquid Chromatography)
Precipitation	Visual inspection

References

1. Sovak M (ed) (1984) Radiocontrast agents. Springer, Berlin Heidelberg New York

2.7 How Are Contrast Media Checked for Freedom from Pyrogens?

B. Wolden

There are two different methods for the testing of possible pyrogens in CM:

1. Rabbit test

This is a qualitative biological test based on the fever response in rabbits. If a pyrogenic substance is injected into a vein of a rabbit, a temperature rise will occur within 3 h.

2. Limulus test

A test sample of CM is incubated with lysate from the blood of the horseshoe crab *(Limulus polyphemus)*. A pyrogenic substance will induce gel formation. This test has been shown to be more sensitive, more rapid and easier to perform than the rabbit test.

2.8 To What Are Colour Changes of Contrast Media Attributable?

D. Herrmann and
B. Wolden

There are two possible reasons for a faint yellow or brown-yellowish discoloration of contrast media solutions:
1. The presence of by-products from the synthesis of the active substance.
2. Chemical decomposition of the active substance or of the by-products; further decomposition beyond deiodination or hydrolysis of the amide structure under the influence of temperature and light.

The yellowish or brown-yellowish discoloration is attributable to organic molecules. As a rule, free inorganic iodine is not detectable within these solutions.

2.9 Does Particulate Contamination Occur, and How Important Is It?

B. Wolden

The significance of particulate contamination in all parenteral products, including CM, has received much attention in recent years. Studies have shown that the proliferation of cells around foreign particles may result in the formation of granulomas in vital organs of the body [1]. Although the size, number and type of particles which can cause toxic effects have not been established, the pharmaceutical industry, medical profession, hospital pharmacists and regulatory agencies all realize the importance of reducing particulate levels in all parenteral products.

Particulate matter may be attributable to different sources, such as raw materials, processing and filling equipment, the container/closure system or environmental contamination. Several methods have been developed for identifying the source of particulates in a product so that they may be eliminated or reduced.

Clarity specifications given in the official monographs (pharmacopoeias like the *United States Pharmacopeia* and the *European Pharmacopoeia*) that should be followed by the pharmaceutical industry state that all bottles/vials for injection should be subjected to visual inspection.

Limits on particulate burden in large-volume parenteral solutions are, for example, 50/ml at 10 µm and 5/ml at 25 µm or 1000/ml at 2.0 µm and 100/ml at 5 µm. These limits apply to the products through to their expiry dates. It should be noted that limits vary between different official monographs/pharmacopoeias and between countries.

References

1. Turco S, David NM (1973) Clinical significance of particulate matter. Hosp Pharm 8:137–140

2.10 Which Factors Reduce the Stability of Contrast Media and What Are the Implications of Storage Recommendations?

D. Hermann

Since the speed of both iodide release and amide saponification depends on temperature, long-term storage of X-ray CM should be at room temperature (15°–25°C). Placing X-ray CM solutions in incubators temporarily, however, in order (Fig. 2.10.1) to warm the solution to body temperature before injection or infusion, does not pose a problem. Figure 2.10.1 shows the iodide release of Ultravist, determined during stability tests involving long-term exposure to heat. The figures make clear that one need have no reservations about storage in incubators for one or more days, or even in water baths warmed to ca. 40°C. Nevertheless, long-term

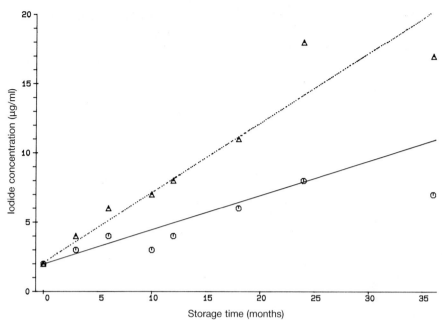

Fig. 2.10.1. Iodide release from Ultravist 370 (50-ml vials) stored at 20°C (▽ −) and 30°C (△ …)

storage at raised temperatures should be avoided.

Putting CM solution in hot water for a short time also produces no problems: for instance, by warming to about 60°–80°C, CM substances that have crystallized when highly concentrated solutions were overly cooled can be redissolved. This addresses a further change that CM solutions may undergo, namely, the purely physical phenomenon of crystallization, which can even occur during transport in winter. It must be borne in mind that highly concentrated CM solutions are usually employed. The concentration normally cited refers to the iodine content: a Urografin solution containing 370 mg I/ml contains 0.66 g diatrizoate meglumine and 0.1 g diatrizoate sodium per ml i.e. a 76% solution! Ultravist 370 contains. 0.769 g iopromide/ml! The X-ray CM Urovison R (100 ml), exclusively made for retrograde pyelography, contains methyl- and propyl-paraben as preservatives, the saturation points of which are exceeded in refrigeration. Finally, aqueous solutions can freeze when put in a freezer. However, as experience has shown not all contents of the bottles in a package crystallize when refrigerated, since this requires seed crystals, and ice starts to form only if the solution is simultaneously shaken. The implication of all of this is that X-ray solutions should preferably be stored at room temperature.

The stability of CM is much more critically affected by continous exposure to light than to heat. Typical light-induced changes are increases in iodide content and decreases in pH, which in ionic CM like Urografin can even lead to the separation of CM acid. Figure 2.10.2 shows the release of iodide from an Ultravist solution as a function of exposure duration at an average workplace illumination of 600 lux.

The speed and extent of light-induced degradation depends greatly on the brightness and spectral composition of the light, since the photochemically active parts of the spectrum are the short-wavelength and near-ultraviolet portions (found in both direct and indirect sunlight). Since these factors are determined by general conditions such as the kind of lighting (natural light, fluorescent lighting, electric lighting) and, in the case of daylight, by the cloud cover and even geographic lo-

cation, no expiration dates for CM can be given for exposure to light. Instead, the expiration dates given refer to storage protected from light. As a general rule of thumb, one day of exposure to an average workplace illumination of 600 lux can be considered unproblematic. Exposure to sunlight should, however, as a rule be avoided, even for short periods since apart from being bright it also includes a considerable proportion of ultraviolet light with especially potent photochemical effects.

The use of brown glass could well improve the stability of CM vis-à-vis exposure to light. However, since CM can be supplied in colourless bottles and used in conditions of normal workplace illumination given a corresponding limitation of shelf life, brown glass may not be used

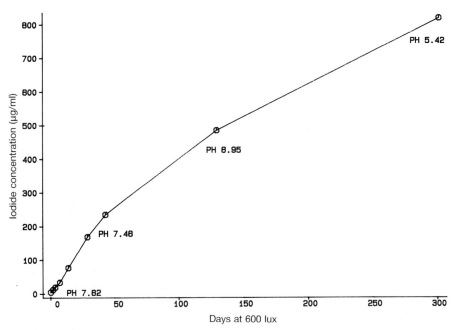

Fig. 2.10.2. Iodide release from 50 ml Ultravist 370 as a function of duration of exposure to 600 lux light

according to the *German Pharmacopoeia,* 9th edn., or the *European Pharmacopoeia:* it is only permitted for extremely light-sensitive pharmaceutical preparations employed parenterally. Since brown glass still lets through a limited amount of radiation in the photochemically active portion of the spectrum, degradation of CM solutions could also still be expected with continuous light exposure, especially in long-term storage where exposure to sunlight cannot be excluded. Thus, even if brown glass is used, it would still be impossible to provide data on stability (expiration dates) given exposure to light.

In addition to short-wave length light, CM can also be damaged by X-rays. For this reason, they must not be stored for long periods in the area of scatter radiation from X-ray apparatus, although one need have no reservations about exposing them for the short periods needed for diagnostic procedures or about preparing them prior to the examination.

2.11 **What Precautions Are Necessary in Drawing Up Contrast Media into Syringes and in Administering Them Using Infusion Devices?**

D. Herrmann

The stopper of a CM bottle should always be pierced using a needle with the narrowest possible lumen and a long bevelled point or with the needle of an infusion unit. Using needles with large lumens, e. g. 2.0 mm, a short bevel, as customarily used in venepuncture, runs the risk of fragmentation, i. e., the punching out of rubber particles. Repeatedly piercing the same spot on the rubber stopper is always to be avoided due to the increased risk of fragmentation. *Nokor* needles (Becton-Dickinson) have proved satisfactory: these are special needles with a scalpel-shaped bevel and a lateral opening. Alternatively, aspiration needles, e. g., *Sterifix* (Braun) are also suitable. Because of the viscosity of CM solutions, the use of special needles or aspiration needles with integrated fluid filters is not possible. On the other hand, an infusion apparatus should always be used with filters, and this mesh filter, usually built into the drip chamber, should permit sufficient rate of fluid flow. Since warming a CM solution to body temperature reduces viscosity by nearly half, drawing it up into a syringe can be made much easier, especially with highly concentrated CM solutions.

X-ray CM interact chemically with synthetic materials, rubber parts, metals and even glass. Because of the variety of characteristics that these materials possess and the synthetic additives that they may contain, only general guidelines can be given in the following.

CM are as a rule compatible with customary disposable administration devices made according to German Industry Standards (DIN) such as disposable plastic syringes (DIN 13098) or infusion devices (DIN 58362). The syringes and/or infusion devices provided by CM manufacturers along with their products have been tested in accordance with such controls.

Glass, stainless steel and chemically neutral synthetics are the preferred materials for reusable devices that can also be cleaned and sterilized prior to use, such as polysulphones for cylindrical cartridges for high-pressure syringes. In general, there are reservations about using drawing-up devices and couplings made of bronze, since reactions such as iodide release can be triggered by the copper ions these give off. On several occasions, discoloration of CM solutions has also been observed after contact with parts made of bronze. If such devices are not made of stainless steel, they must be completely and faultlessly chrome plated, both internally and externally.

2.12 How Long Do Contrast Media Remain Usable After the Original Container Has Been Opened?

D. Herrmann

In general, any CM solution not used in the course of an examination should be discarded. As a working figure for the maximum time for which CM can be used the original container has been opened or it has been transferred into delivery system, a period of 4 h should not be exceeded. After longer periods, there is an increasing danger of microbial or bacterial growth and a pyrogenic reaction. During this time, crystallization due to evaporative loss can also occur: seed crystals can form on the surface of the liquid exposed to the air and this could then induce immediate crystallization of the entire contents of the bottle. The danger of light-induced degradation also exists.

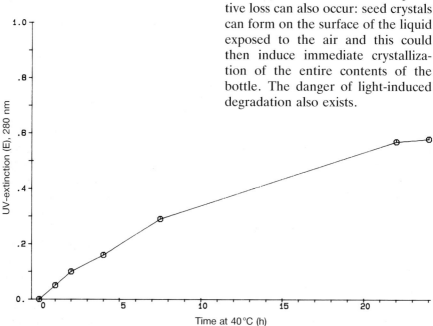

Fig. 2.12.1. Global migration from X-ray CM syringes showing the rise in ultraviolet extinction in water for injection

If an injection solution is left standing for several hours in a disposable syringe, it can take up vulcanization additives from the piston stopper, resulting in an additional insult to the patient. Figure 2.12.1 shows the increase in ultraviolet extinction resulting from migration of an elastomer additive.

cluded in, for example, the *United States Pharmacopeia,* 22nd edn.

Mixing CM with other drugs should only be done after testing the compatibility of the CM with the drug in question; such mixtures should be prepared immediately before administration. For the reasons mentioned in Sect. 2.12, sterilizing mixtures for the purpose of saving them should be avoided.

2.13 May Contrast Media Be Diluted or Mixed with Other Drugs?

D. Hermann

This question must first be considered in terms of drug regulations. By diluting or mixing CM with other preparations, new drugs are produced, and the hospital pharmacist, for example, must take responsibility for them. This also holds for mixtures with standard infusion solutions. For purposes of injection, the preferred choice for dilution is a physiological salt solution or, depending on the desired osmotic pressure, water. The compatibility with other solutions can basically be judged by colour, cloudiness and pH. One should not go outside the pH range defined by the quality specification of the CM, e.g. in the case of Ultravist, outside the pH range 6.5–8.0. Because of the possible inducement of iodide release, mixing CM with solutions that have strongly reducing effects or with preparations containing heavy metals should be avoided. Special analytical chemistry methods are in-

2.14 Is the Resterilization and Reuse of Disposable Angiography Catheters Justified?

M. Thelen

Definition and Legal Situation

The reprocessing and resterilization of disposable material has been the subject of controversial discussion for some time now. For economic reasons, many users have long since started to resterilize expensive disposable materials such as intravascular catheters and measuring probes. These articles come under Article 2, Section 1a, of the German Drug Law, which states that "medical, dental or veterinary instruments, where they are intended for once-only use and where it is clear from the labelling that they have been subjected to a process for reducing the germ count", are regarded as drugs. However, the designation "disposable article" is the concern of the manufacturer – there is no such

definition in law – and, in general, reprocessing or resterilisation is not regarded as manufacturing in the sense of the German Drug Law (Article 4, Section 14). It is not forbidden by law. Thus, this issue is not explicitly regulated by the law.

A comment by the German Federal Office of Health reads as follows (Federal Health Bulletin 31, Number 9/88, page 343):

By their very name, disposable articles are conceived for just a single use. This is apparent even from the choice of the materials used. The plastics employed are usually heat sensitive. The types of synthetic materials used are so varied that the user will hardly be in a position to recognize the extent to which the usability of an article is impaired by repeated use, repeated processing and repeated sterilization. The articles must not only be functional, they must also be free from impurities of a mechanical, chemical and biological nature and must also be capable of being sterilized without being damaged. Anyone who uses disposable articles several times does this on his own responsibility.

According to DIN 58953, Part 8, the processing and renewed sterilization of disposable articles is considered inadmissible: "because material damage might occur as a result of the processing and/or resterilization which could then jeopardize safe use of the disposable article."

Similarly, the resterilization of disposable materials is rejected according to the recommendations of the Centers for Disease Control (CDC Guidelines 1985):

Articles and materials which cannot be cleaned, sterilized or disinfected without altering their physical integrity and function should not be sterilized. Reprocessing measures leading to toxic byproducts or which impair the safety or effectiveness of the article or material should be avoided.

The recommendations and norms quoted above are not legally binding, but it should be noted as regards their legal quality that they are recommendations which reflect the present state of science and technology.

Reprocessing of Disposable Angiography Catheters

In any reprocessing procedure it is necessary that each individual step be carefully validated, and the cleansing, sterilization and material safety must be checked individually. Detailed quality criteria must be established for each of these steps. Apart from questions of sterility and the physical and functional properties of the catheters, attention is drawn here in particular to the toxicological safety with interactions between catheter materials and cleansing agents and disinfectants. No such validated quality criteria exist at the present time.

Given the plethora of materials and combinations of materials, and the variety of shapes and diameters in which catheters come, as well as the likewise innumerable number of cleansing agents and disinfectants, it is therefore doubtful whether reprocessing – regardless of its technical feasibility – is economically expedient. No balance of the costs which takes account of all these aspects, including the equipment to be acquired and the resulting personnel and environmental costs, is so far available.

Another aspect must be taken into consideration if the catheters which are used in angiographic examinations are to be used again. All catheters have thrombogenic properties and promote blood clotting, a phenomenon which is related to the smoothness of the material used for the catheter. To date no study has been conducted to investigate whether electrical charges developing on the surface of the catheter may enhance the risk of thrombosis. We do know from Kido's report (see [1] in Sect. 2.15) that the passage of a guidewire through a catheter causes considerable surface damage, so that an increase in thrombogenicity seems certain. Therefore, caution is advised when reusing catheters in angiography to avoid the increased risk of thromboembolism.

There is no law against recycling angiographic catheters; however, besides economic concerns, there are so many other problems involved, especially ones pertaining to quality control, that such processing would have to be delegated to central recycling plants. Presently, no quality control criteria exist for cleaning, sterilization, and functional and chemical integrity, and since there are also indications that thrombus development may be promoted by recycling, recycled catheters should not be used in angiographic procedures.

2.15 Is There an Increased Risk of Coagulation when Catheters Are Reused?

P. Dawson

Aside from the considerations outlined in Sect. 2.14, there is another aspect to be considered when catheters are reused for angiography. All catheters are thrombogenic and activate blood coagulation on contact. The phenomenon is a function of the material used and of its surface finish. No data are available on possible changes occurring in the thrombogenicity of catheter materials undergoing sterilization procedures. One thing is, however, known from the work of Kido et al. [1], namely that the passage of a guidewire through a catheter is likely to produce considerable surface damage to an extent that an increase in thrombogenicity seems certain. Caution is urged in the reuse of catheters for angiography to avoid an increase in the risk of thromboembolic accidents.

References

1. Kido DK, King PK, Manziona JV, Simon JH (1988) The role of catheters and guidewires in the production of angiographic thromboembolic complications. Invest Radiol 23:S359–S364

CHAPTER 3

Influence of Contrast Media on Organs and Vessels

3.1 What Are the Mechanisms of Toxicity Associated with Contrast Media?

P. Dawson

Three factors are usually cited as involved in CM toxicity, namely hyperosmolality, chemotoxicity and charge, although strictly speaking charge should be incorporated under the heading "chemotoxicity" since it forms part of that phenomenon.

Hyperosmolality effects are quite easily understood in general terms. They include acute expansion of the plasma volume, generalized vasodilatation resulting from an effect on smooth muscle, rigidification of red cells, histamine release from basophils and mast cells and endothelial injury, which may lead to thrombophlebitis or frank thrombosis following venous injection. These hyperosmolality phenomena are all due to the nonspecific effects of the highly concentrated solutions of the formulations in clinical use.

Chemotoxic effects arise from the properties of the CM molecules themselves. These are less easy to understand and have only been unravelled in the last decade or so. A stimulus and a help in elucidating the processes was the arrival of the newer generation of nonionic CM

since having molecules with different detailed structures and different magnitudes of chemotoxicity provided an experimental test bed for investigation.

In summary, it seems that chemotoxic effects are mediated by nonspecific interactions between CM molecules and biological macromolecules. While some hydrophilic interactions are undoubtedly possible, it seems likely, since the hydrophilic portions of the CM molecules are solvated in water solution, that most of the interactions are between hydrophobic groups. The hydrophobic groups of any CM molecule are, most importantly, the benzene ring and iodine central core of the molecule. These hydrophobic interactions are augmented by Coulomb interactions when charged ions are involved, as in the case of the conventional agents.

The route to minimizing chemotoxic interactions therefore lies in eliminating charge and in masking the hydrophobic core of such molecules by an array of hydrophilic moieties. This prescription is essentially a description of the current nonionic agents. These, by definition, lack charge and all have an extensive array of hydrophilic groups around the hydrophobic core. It is true that these hydrophilic groups were designed to restore high water solubility lost when the carboxyl group of the ionic CM was eliminated, but they have had the serendipitous effect of also meeting the design specification now understood in general terms for an agent with low chemotoxicity. The current generation of nonionic agents differ, of course, in detailed structure and have been shown to differ in degree of toxicity in laboratory studies, though there is no evidence of significant differences between them in manifest clinical toxicity.

Insights of this kind may lead to the rational design of better contrast agents using computer design techniques.

References

1. Dawson P (1984) Chemotoxicity of contrast media and clinical adverse effects: a review. Invest Radiol 20:583–591
2. Howell MJ, Dawson P (1985) Contrast agents and enzyme inhibition. II Mechanisms. Br J Radiol 58:845–848

3.2 Do Contrast Media Affect the Viscosity of Blood?

N. H. Strickland

The viscosity of any cell system, including blood (a plasma-red cell system), is affected by four major factors: the suspending phase viscosity, the cellular size, the cellular deformability and the presence of aggregates, which in the case of blood are red cell rouleaux, that is, red cell aggregates induced by plasma proteins. CM alter blood viscosity by affecting these four parameters to a greater or lesser degree.

The viscosity of liquids may be simply and reliably calculated from their shear rate using a bob-in-cup viscometer apparatus. All neat CM behave as true Newtonian fluids since their viscosity does not vary with shear rate [4]. Experiments examining how various concentrations of CM affect the viscosity of the suspending phase of blood (i.e. plasma) show that the viscosities of all plasma-CM mixtures are very high in comparison with plasma. Mixtures with the ionic monomer ioxaglate showed lower viscosities than mixtures with corresponding concentrations of ionic or nonionic monomeric CM. Mixtures of CM with isotonic phosphate-buffered saline behaved similarly to the plasma-CM mixtures [5]. This is important because it demonstrates that CM do not significantly affect the plasma proteins and in particular they do not cause appreciable plasma protein aggregation or precipitation.

Numerous studies have demonstrated that the hyperosmolality of CM reduces cellular size. This is reflected in the reduction in blood haematocrit engendered by CM and can be explained solely by the hypertonicity of the suspending phase of the mixture [5].

In addition, different CM alter red cell morphology to varying degrees, causing some erythrocytes to lose their normal biconcave shape and form echinocytes. Light microscopy and scanning electron microscopy [1] have shown that the ionic dimer ioxaglate results in only slight changes in red cell morphology compared with equivalent concentrations of ionic and nonionic mono-meric CM. This phenomenon cannot be attributed merely to the osmolality of the solution since it has been shown that changes in red cell morphology engendered by the highest concentrations of ioxaglate studied (75%) were less than those produced by hyperosmolar saline [1].

The viscosity characteristics of red cell suspensions in the presence of different concentrations of CM are largely influenced by the additional effects of the CM upon cellular deformability and the presence of red cell rouleaux. The experimental situation is simpler at high shear rates (≤ 128.5 s^{-1}) because the effects of the small cellular aggregation forces then become negligible, so rouleaux can be ignored.

At low shear rates cellular aggregation forces become significant, so rouleaux will significantly affect viscosity measurements. At low shear rates (≥ 0.277 s^{-1}) viscosity falls rapidly with increasing concentration for all types of CM. This fall in viscosity at low shear is due to cellular aggregation decreasing at higher CM concentrations, so the suspension becomes less viscous. CM can inhibit cellular aggregation in at least two ways. First, a direct effect on the red cell inhibits rouleaux formation. Second, the viscosity of the suspending phase increases as the CM concentration increases and this produces higher local shear forces in the red cells, tending to pull the cellular aggregates apart.

It has been shown that at both high and low shear rates, the rate of change of viscosity with CM concentration differs markedly between the various types of CM [2,5]. The con-ventional ionic monomers caused most disturbance to blood viscosity. The monoacid dimer ioxaglate was least disturbing to the viscometric characteristics of blood and the newer, nonionic monomers were intermediate in their effects. This is surprising because, in contradistinction to the accepted hierarchy for the effects of CM at the molecular level [3], ioxaglate is closest to the ideal of total inertness with respect to changes in viscometric properties of red cell suspensions. The explanation for this observation must at present be speculative, but it seems likely that what matters most in determining low viscometric disturbance for a CM is low osmolality, low density and low inherent viscosity, rather than its ionic or nonionic status.

Clinical Significance of Changes in Viscosity

Once uniform distribution of, for example, a 50-ml bolus of CM has taken place in the whole circulation, the final low plasma concentration of about 2% will have very little effect on blood viscosity. However, during in vivo angiographic procedures there are a number of situations in which very high concentrations of CM are present. These high concentrations can be expected to have significant effects on blood rheology because of the resulting high density, osmolality and viscosity.

Early after bolus injection of CM into large vessels, mixing between it and blood is incomplete. Blood cells at the CM-blood interface will be in contact with very high concentrations of CM and this may cause marked rheological effects; results predict that where shear rate is high, along the walls of vessels and at the origin of side branches, viscosity will be increased [4].

After selective injection into any organ, there will be high local CM concentration in its microcirculation and this may be expected to alter the normal rheology of the organ's microvasculature. In small vessels where shear rate is high the increased viscosity of blood exposed to high CM concentrations could lead to increased sludging and occlusion of these small vessels. In other small vessels where shear rate is low, the decreased viscosity of blood in contact with high CM concentrations may increase the flow through these vessels. Differential perfusion of the microvascular bed may thus result and this would not be an accurate representation of the normal pattern of blood flow through those vessels in the absence of CM. Such effects could be accentuated by the initial nonuniform distribution of the injected CM within the vascular bed.

A final important clinical situation is created during an angioplasty procedure. Blood flow around the angioplasty site may be reduced almost to zero in the presence of atheromatous plaque and an intraluminal balloon catheter or laser. This will accentuate the rheological effects of high bolus concentrations of CM delivered locally, with repercussions on haemodynamics. The nature of such changes will depend upon whether the prevailing local shear forces are high or low. During a balloon or laser angioplasty procedure the stasis itself would be expected to produce conditions favouring low shear forces, which should lower blood viscosity in the presence of high CM concentrations, and this might, if anything, be beneficial. However, local shear forces are more likely to be high if a rotary atherectomy device is used, or in the immediate postangioplasty situation where high flow conditions are reinstated and in addition a local contrast bolus is injected at the angioplasty site to document the radiographic result. The increase in viscosity under such circumstances might favour thrombus formation on a freshly cracked plaque or in the distal run-off vessels.

References

1. Aspelin P (1978) Effect of ionic and non-ionic contrast media on morphology of human erythrocytes. Acta Radiol Diagn 19:675–687
2. Hardeman NR, Goedhart P, Koeni Y (1991) The effect of low-osmolar ionic and non-ionic contrast media on human blood viscosity, erythrocyte morphology, and aggregation behaviour. Invest Radiol 26:810–818
3. Howell L, Dawson P (1986) Contrast agents and enzyme inhibition. II Mechanisms. Br J Radiol 59:987–991
4. Strickland NH, Rampling MW, Dawson P, Martin G (1992) Contrast media-induced effects on blood rheology and their importance in angiography. Clin Radiol (in press)
5. Strickland NH, Rampling MW, Dawson P, Martin G (1992) The effects of radiocontrast media on the rheological properties of blood. Eur J Haemorheol (in press)

3.3 Are There any Differences Between Ionic and Nonionic Contrast Media in Their Effect on Coagulation?

P. Dawson

All the available evidence supports the idea that iodinated intravascular CM are qualitatively similar in their effects on coagulation and differ only in the magnitude of these effects [2]. Thus, both nonionics and ionics interfere with the coagulation cascade at a number of levels, in particular inhibiting fibrin polymerization and inhibiting platelet aggregation. The nonionics, however, have significantly weaker effects, particularly at higher concentrations, than do the ionic agents of conventional or low osmolality. The occasional formation in syringes or catheters of clots during angiographic procedures carried out with the less anticoagulant nonionic agents [4] has been misinterpreted in some quarters as evidence for some "procoagulant" property of these materials. Indeed, the adjective "thrombogenic" has been applied to them. There is, however, absolutely no evidence on which to base such an idea. Some statements, made in good faith and intended to be helpful, to the effect that prolonged contact between nonionic agents and blood should be avoided, are also misleading. Certainly, angiographic procedures should be carried out as quickly as is compatible with other aspects of safety, but there is no question but that nonionic agents

are also anticoagulant and are therefore entirely helpful in preventing coagulation and subsequent thromboembolic events [3]. They are simply somewhat less helpful in this sense than the ionic agents.

It is also important to realize that the lesser anticoagulant properties of the nonionic agents are part and parcel of their generally greater inertness and biocompatibility [1]. More anticoagulant CM are more toxic.

The role played by catheter and syringe materials in promoting coagulation by contact activation is just as important as the role of contrast agents in inhibiting it. There are significant differences between materials: for instance, glass is a much more powerful activator than any plastic and polyurethane tends to be a more powerful activator than polyethylene [3].

In principle, a more careful angiographic technique might arguably be necessary in clinical angiography with nonionic agents than with ionic agents but, on the basis of extensive experience over several years in Europe, there appears to be no significant difference in the incidence of problems in practice with the new, and in other regards better and safer, agents.

References

1. Dawson P (1985) Chemotoxicity of contrast agents and clinical adverse effects. Invest Radiol 20:584–591
2. Dawson P et al (1986) Contrast, coagulation and fibrinolysis. Invest Radiol 21:248–252
3. Dawson P, Strickland NS (1991) Thromboembolic phenomena in clinical

angiography: role of materials and technique. JVIR 2:125–132

4. Robertson MJF (1987) Blood clot formation in angiographic syringes containing non-ionic contrast media. Radiology 162:621–622

3.4 Do Contrast Media Affect Cardiovascular Function?

P. Dawson

CM have a variety of adverse effects on the cardiovascular system [5]. They have primary central effects on the heart – myocardial contractility, electrophysiology and coronary blood flow are all affected – and primary effects on the peripheral vasculature. They also expand plasma volume [6], adversely affect blood rheology [3] and have anticoagulant properties [4]. Homeostatic responses are invoked and, although at first sight entirely physiologically appropriate, these may not in some patients be entirely desirable.

One of the most stressful events when a large bolus of CM is delivered into the intravascular space by any route is the generalized vasodilatation engendered, which results in systemic hypotension with a reflex tachycardia [5]. This is largely a hyperosmolality-mediated effect on smooth muscle, but inhibition of acetylcholine in blood and tissues [2] and histamine release [1] have also been invoked as mediators.

The effects on the heart itself are obviously greatest when injection is directly into the coronary arteries, as during coronary arteriography. There are marked depressant effects on cardiac pump function, however assessed, which are dose-dependent and most persistent in the ischaemic heart. They are also cumulative, hence the need for rest intervals between injections in clinical work. Osmolality, chemotoxicity, oxygen displacement and ionic content all contribute to these effects [5].

There are also striking changes in electrophysiology following coronary artery injection [5]. These are due to a combination of direct and indirect neurally mediated effects on sinus rate, intracardiac conduction velocity, duration of ventricular depolarization-repolarization processes and a consequent liability to tachyarrhythmias. The ventricular fibrillation threshold is reduced in a dose-dependent fashion.

Coronary blood flow is also increased by CM [5]. This is not, as would first appear, a necessarily desirable consequence of their injection in that the hyperaemic response occurs in more normal areas of vascularity but not in areas of abnormal vascularity. There may, therefore, be a steal phenomenon rendering the ischaemic areas even more ischaemic.

The nonionic agents are also associated with all these effects, but to a markedly lesser degree. Indeed, in some animal studies they have, rather than a negative inotropic effect, a small positive inotropic effect. The differences are based on their lower osmolality, their lower chemotoxicity and their almost insignificant capacity for binding calcium [5].

References

1. Assem ESK, Bray K, Dawson P (1983) The release of histamine from human basophils by radiological contrast agents. Br J Radiol 56:647–652
2. Dawson P, Edgerton D (1983) Contrast media and enzyme inhibition. I Acetylcholinesterase. Br J Radiol 56:653–656
3. Dawson P, Harrison MJG, Weisblat E (1983) Effect of contrast media on red cell filtrability and morphology. Br J Radiol 56:707–710
4. Dawson P et al (1986) Contrast, coagulation and fibrinolysis. Invest Radiol 21:248–252
5. Dawson P (1989) Cardiovascular effects of contrast agents. Am J Cardiol 64:2E–9E
6. Hine AL, Lui D, Dawson P (1985) Contrast media osmolality and plasma volume changes. Acta Radiol 26:753–756

3.5 Do Contrast Media Affect Pulmonary Function?

P. Dawson

There is no doubt that in a number of ways various contrast procedures may affect pulmonary function, though it must be said that this is an area in which detailed study has been lacking.

When hyperosmolar CM are delivered directly into the bronchial tree, osmotic effects may produce acute pulmonary oedema [4].

When Lipiodol is used for lymphography the CM finds it way through the thoracic duct into the subclavian vein and hence through the right side of the heart and into the lungs. Globules of CM are trapped in the capillaries and may be seen on chest radiographs. In the period the lungs are dealing with this oil there is impairment of lung function, with a reduction in pulmonary compliance and decreases in pulmonary capillary blood volume and pulmonary diffusion capacity [4].

In bronchography, as might be expected, the introduction of CM into the tracheobronchial tree causes some degree of breathlessness. Measurements of vital capacity and maximum breathing capacity show an average reduction of 20% immediately following unilateral bronchography and 30% in the case of bilateral bronchography [8]. Diffusion scans with macro-aggregates of albumin carried out an hour or so after bronchography may show localized diffusion defects in the lungs [8], presumably in response to partial bronchial obstruction by CM. Ventilation scans also show areas of deficit [3]. There is a significant reduction in diffusion capacity, which may not return to normal for 72 h. Not surprisingly, direct introduction of CM of the bronchial tree may also precipitate bronchospasm, particularly in asthmatic patients [1].

As regards intravascular contrast agents, Littner et al. demonstrated that subclinical bronchospasm could be routinely detected in patients receiving peripheral venous boluses of CM in urography-type doses [5]. Dawson et al. confirmed this observation and noted that there were smaller changes when a nonionic CM was used [3]. It seems reasonable to suggest, though relevant convincing clinical studies have not been carried out, that nonionic CM should be used in all patients at risk for bronchospasm. This would include not only asthmatics per se but also those with chronic obstructive airways disease with an element of bronchospasm.

Another observation of interest is that occasional cases of noncardiogenic, acute pulmonary oedema based on increased capillary permeability may occasionally be seen following intravenous CM administration [2]. The increased permeability may be based on vascular injury by the CM and/or the release of histamine in the histamine-rich pulmonary bed. Interestingly, intravenous injection of ionic CM has been shown to increase pulmonary capillary permeability routinely and to cause a marked, if transitory, elevation for extravascular lung water [6]. A nonionic CM has been demonstrated to engender much less marked effects and pretreatment with methylprednisolone [7] significantly reduces this experimental subclinical pulmonary oedema. Detailed studies have not been made, but these changes probably affect diffusion and compliance.

References

1. Beales JSM, Saxton HM (1968) The radiographic demonstration of bronchospasm and its relief by aminophylline. Br J Radiol 41:899–901
2. Chambalin WH, Stockman GD, Wray WP (1979) Shock and non cardiogenic pulmonary oedema following meglumine diatrizoate for intravenous urography. Am J Med 67:684–686
3. Dawson P, Pitfield J, Britton J (1983) Contrast media and bronchospasm: a study with iopamidol. Clin Radiol 34:227–230
4. Gold WH (1965) Pulmonary function abnormalities after lymphangiography. N Engl J Med 273:519–524
5. Littner MR, Rosenfield AT, Ulreich S, Putman CE (1977) Evaluation of bronchospasm during excretion urography. Radiology 124:17–21
6. Mare K, Violante M, Zack A (1984) Contrast media induced pulmonary oedema. Comparison of ionic and non-ionic agents in an animal model. Invest Radiol 19:566–569
7. Mare K, Violante M, Zack A (1985) Pulmonary oedema following high intravenous doses of diatrizoate in the rat. Effects of corticosteroid pretreatment. Acta Radiol 26:477–482
8. Suprenant E, Wilson A, Bennett L, O'Reilly R, Webber M (1968) Changes in regional pulmonary function following bronchography. Radiology 91:736–741

3.6 Do Contrast Media Affect Hepatic Function?

V. Taenzer

There are scarcely any reports on the effects of the administration of intravascular CM on hepatic function. In studies of pigs, only slight statistically nonsignificant changes in the hepatic enzymes were observed after administration of both ionic (Metrizoate 370) and nonionic substances (iohexol 370) in relatively high doses for selective coeliac angiography with a balloon occlusion of the coeliac trunk.

Further experimental studies of the tolerability of uroangiographic X-ray CM in Wistar rats with cirrhosis of the liver showed that marked worsening of measures of cirrhosis occurred after administration of both ionic and nonionic X-ray CM.

Even in patients with healthy livers, the use of ionic and nonionic substances for visceral angiography results in slight temporary increases in hepatic enzymes. The maximum increase in liver enzymes (alkaline phosphatase, glutamate pyruvate transaminase, glutamate oxaloacetate transaminase) is seen between 48 and 72 h after CM administration.

By contrast, in double-blind studies of intravenous ionic and nonionic renal CM for both urography and digital subtraction angiography, no significant changes in the liver enzymes were demonstrated. These liver-specific parameters were also not affected in patients with healthy livers when intravenous cholangiographic CM were administered and measurements made prior to and up to 3 days after CM administration.

3.7 Do Contrast Media Affect Renal Function?

J. E. Scherberich

Water-soluble X-ray CM are basically safe pharmaceutical preparations with a wide range of uses. Nevertheless, all CM are nephrotoxic to greater or lesser degree [1–3]. "Nephrotoxicity" is defined as a (usually temporary) increase in serum creatinine concentration of at least 0.5–1 mg/dl or as a drop in creatinine clearance of at least 25%; however, a number of definitions may be found in the literature on the subject. The acute reduction in kidney function peaks sometime around the 4th–7th day after CM administration; there then follows a slow phase of repair lasting 1–4 weeks, which is accompanied by a normalization of serum creatinine.

The frequency of CM-induced acute kidney failure is about 0.6% (i.v. urography) in outpatients with healthy kidneys and ca. 4%–5% (angiography) in hospitalized patients with healthy kidneys. CM trigger nephropathy much more frequently in patients with diabetic nephropathy ($\geq 70\%$) or pre-existing kidney disease (about 22%), and on repeated administration [1–5]. Most CM-induced kidney damage is temporary and asymptomatic; however, acute kidney failure also occurs. According to prospective studies, CM seem to be involved in 12% of all cases of acute kidney failure in hospitalized patients [1–3]. There are recognized predisposing factors (see Sects. 4.8–4.12). It is more difficult to predict the course of oliguria/anuria than that of polyuria.

The pathogenesis of CM-related nephrotoxicity is not yet completely understood. Important factors, however, may include [4–7, 11]:

1. Disturbances of glomerular microcirculation
   - pH, electrical charge, osmolality, chemotoxicity of the CM
   - Sludging of erythrocytes
   - Pseudoagglutination (CM and para-/cryoglobulinaemia)
   - Negative effect on glomerular ultrafiltration coefficient.
2. "Biphasic" alterations in renal haemodynamics
   - Initial vasodilatation and subsequent vasoconstriction

- Reduction of glomerular filtration rate (GFR) with largely unchanged renal plasma flow
- Intrarenal activation of the renin-angiotensin II system.
3. Alterations of medullary perfusion
   - For example, corticomedullary shunts are found experimentally.
4. Direct tubulotoxic effects
   - Intracytoplasmic vacuole formation.
   - Shedding of the brush border in the lumen of the proximal tubules with the formation of so-called obstructing blebs, which aggregate and block the lumen.
   - Disturbed or reduced Na^+ reabsorption in the proximal tubule ("Thurau mechanism"), leading to high end-distal Na^+ concentration, which triggers, via the macula densa, the release of intrarenal renin-angiotensin II and decreases in GFR
   - Intracellular Ca^{2+} accumulation
   - Increase in oxygen free radicals
   - Instability of the cytoskeleton
   - Suppression of Na^+, K^+-ATPase (CM chemotoxicity).
   - Aggregation of CM with Bence Jones proteins or Tamm-Horsfall mucoproteins.

Sensitive measures of CM-induced renal impairment include: creatinine clearance, serum α_1-microglobulin, and the levels of "major tubular enzymes" in urine. Since alterations of the tubule are the most important pathophysiological effects, epithelial membrane proteins such as alanine aminopeptidase, alkaline phospha-tase, and γ-glutamyl transpeptidase are especially suitable parameters [7, 8]. In contrast, the frequently favoured β-N-acetyl-D-glucosaminidase (referred to as β-NAG) has only low sensitivity as a measure of CM-induced tubulotoxicity.

In patients with kidney disease the more serious the impairment of kidney function, the greater the risk that the further reduction in renal function induced by CM will not remain temporary and asymptomatic. Acute renal failure can result. The first clinical signs are polyuria or oligoanuria and radiologically persistent signs are seen on nephrography. The following symptoms are observed in succession: oedema, increase in weight, fatigue, dysponea caused by pulmonary oedema, possibly hyperventilation, presternal pains, muscular weakness, fasciculation, pruritis, tendency to bleed, convulsions and coma.

In pathogenetic terms, there are various possible mechanisms of CM-related nephrotoxicity that can trigger acute kidney failure. Understandably, their effects on an already functionally impaired kidney are usually much graver than on a healthy organ.

References

1. Bahlmann J, Krüskemper HL (1973) Elimination of iodine-containing contrast media by haemodialysis. Nephron 10:250–254
2. Berns AS (1989) Nephrotoxicity of contrast media. Kidney Int 36:730–740
3. Dawson P (1987) Aspects of contrast media nephrotoxicity. In: Felix R et al (eds) Contrast media, from the past to the future. Thieme, Stuttgart, pp 137–148

4. Golman K, Almén T (1985) Contrast media-induced nephrotoxicity. Survey and present state. Invest Radiol 20:92–97
5. Kumar S, Muchmore A (1990) Tamm-Horsfall Protein-Uromodulin. Kidney Int 37:1395–1401
6. Neumayer H-H, Junge W, Küfner A, Wenning A (1989) Prevention of radiocontrast-media induced nephrotoxicity by the calcium channel blocker nitrendipine: a prospective randomised clinical trial. Nephrol Dial Transplant 4:1030–1036
7. Scherberich JE (1989) Immunological and ultrastructural analysis of shedding of tubular membrane-bound enzymes in urine of patients with kidney diseases. Clin Chim Acta 185:271–282
8. Scherberich J, Tuengerthal S, Kollath J (1983) Monitoring of contrast media nephrotoxicity by specific kidney tissue proteinuria of membrane antigens. In: Taenzer W, Zeitler E (eds) CM in urography. Thieme, Stuttgart, pp 37–42
9. Scherberich JE, Wolf G, Albers C et al (1989) Glomerular and tubular membrane antigens reflecting cellular adaptation in human renal failure. Kidney Int 36, S 27:38–51
10. Schwab SJ, Hlatky MA, Pieper KS et al (1989) Contrast media nephrotoxicity: a randomized controlled trial of a nonionic and an ionic radiographic contrast agent. N Engl J Med 320:149–153
11. Scherberich JE, Rautschka E, Fischer A, Kollath J, Riemann J (1991) Tubular histuria: Clinical evaluation of the different nephrotoxic potential of x-ray contrast media. Contrib Nephrol (im Druck)
12. Taenzer W, Wende A (eds) (1989) Recent developments in nonionic contrast media. Thieme, Stuttgart
13. Taenzer W, Zeitler E (eds) (1983) Contrast media in urography, angiography and computerized tomography. Thieme, Stuttgart
14. Vari RC, Natarajan LA, Whitescarver SA, Jackson BA, Ott CE (1988) Induction, prevention and mechanisms of contrast media-induced acute renal failure. Kidney Int 33:399–707

3.8 Do Iodinated X-Ray Contrast Media Affect Thyroid Function?

B. Glöbel

Iodinated X-ray CM do not have any direct influence on thyroid function. Nevertheless, the preparations do contain small amounts of free iodide. Moreover, after the CM is introduced into the living organism, iodide splits off from the molecule. Both free and separated-off iodide take part in iodine metabolism and can influence thyroid function in this way. Iodide in amounts exceeding the normal daily intake can lead to a decrease in hormone synthesis (Plummer's treatment, Wolff-Chaikoff effect). In latent hyperthyroidism, where an iodine deficiency has prevented the condition from becoming clinically manifest, the iodide can be sufficient to trigger manifest hyperthyroidism.

The engendering of hypofunction is primarily a risk in newborns and small children, where relatively high iodide concentrations are reached because of the comparatively small volume of distribution in these patients. The effects of iodinated X-ray CM are generally reversible, however, and subside once the iodide has been excreted. Hyperthyroidism is mainly a risk for older individuals. The real risk here is in fact that a hyperthyroid metabolic condition could progress into a so-called thyrotoxic crisis. With present knowledge, there is no screening test enabling recognition of the risk of thyrotoxic crisis in advance. The incidence of thyrotoxic crisis is estimated to be about 1 : 50,000 in Germany, independent of the source of the increased iodine supply.

3.9 What Is the Relationship Between Iodinated Contrast Media and the Blood-Brain Barrier?

P. Dawson

The water-soluble agents, especially the nonionic agents with their high hydrophilicity, penetrate the central nervous system very poorly because of the existence of the blood-brain barrier. It is for this reason that normal brain enhances poorly on CM administration. However, there are regions such as the pituitary gland where the blood-brain barrier is absent and CM may enter freely. In any case, when injected in high concentrations directly into the cerebral vessels, the agents themselves may cause significant injury and disruption to the blood-brain barrier, thereby effecting an entry into the central nervous system. High osmolality plays a role in this, but neurotoxicity does not correlate well with osmolality of the agent and it is clear that other factors such as chemotoxicity play a significant part both in the blood-brain barrier injury and, of course, in subsequent neurotoxic events.

Penetration through the blood-brain barrier is dose dependent and appears to be a function of the plasma/cerebrospinal fluid concentration gradient. The degree of penetration correlates well with toxic manifestations. It has been found that the cerebrospinal fluid concentration of an ionic CM 1 h after intravenous injection was approximately 1.5% of the initial blood concentration. Given the great sensitivity of neural tissues, it seems reasonable to consider a role for neurotoxicity in the so-called systemic adverse reactions to CM.

Possible protective measures against neurotoxic effects have been explored. Pretreatment with steroids and low molecular weight Dextran, alone or in combination, have proved efficacious in reducing neurotoxicity. Steroid pretreatment apparently reduces penetration of CM into the central nervous system even after injury to the blood-brain barrier. It is known that neurotoxic effects are greater in patients with defects of the blood-brain barrier and in patients with high plasma levels of CM. The neuroprotective effects of steroids have been postulated to form the basis for their claimed protective effects against major adverse reactions. However, the use of intrathecal corticosteroids to reduce arachnoiditis, paradoxically, promotes its development.

3.10 Do Contrast Media Affect the Central Nervous System?

M. R. Sage

Introduction

Depending on the nature of the examination, intraarterial, intravenous or intrathecal injections of water-soluble CM are made during certain neuroimaging procedures. As a result, CM comes into contact with at least one of the three interfaces of the CNS, namely the blood-brain interface (BBB), the blood-cerebrospinal fluid (CSF) interface or the brain-CSF interface [5]. Potentially this could result in neurotoxicity. In general the overall toxicity of nonionic. CM is less than that of equivalent iodine concentrations of ionic CM [6].

Neuroangiography

Neurotoxicity is a recognized complication of cerebral and spinal angiography [6]. Many of the neurological complications of cerebral angiography are probably related to the catherization procedure rather than the CM [3]. Other complications may result from the haemodynamic effects of CM such as hypotension, bradycardia, vasodilation or vasospasm, alterations in regional cerebral blood flow and an increase in blood viscosity and aggregation and clumping of red blood cells [2, 6, 8].

In general, these haemodynamic effects are less marked with nonionic CM.

The actual role of CM itself in neurological complications is not clear. During neuroangiography, CM comes in contact with the endothelium of the cerebral or spinal cord capillaries. The morphological characteristics of neural endothelium differ from those of non-neural capillaries. The neural endothelium behaves like a plasma membrane [1], controlling the passage of many substances, including water-soluble molecules, between blood and brain and hence maintaining the homeostasis of the neurons [5]. This constitutes the so-called blood-brain barrier (BBB) [6]. An intact BBB therefore prevents the CM from coming into direct contact with the nervous tissue itself by preventing the passage of the CM from the blood into the extracellular fluid of the brain or spine. The integrity of the BBB is therefore probably the major factor in preventing neurotoxicity of intravascular CM. When the BBB is deliberately broken down with hypertonic mannitol, seizures have been observed [6] and seizures may be provoked during neuroangiography if there is a pathological breakdown in the BBB [6]. The pathological loss of the integrity of the BBB allows the CM to cross into the external fluid of the brain, resulting in a direct chemotoxic effect. Similarly, hypertonic CM injected intra-arterially may themselves increase the permeability of the BBB [5, 6] and therefore allow the passage of such CM into the extracellular fluid of the brain. As ionic CM are more hypertonic than corresponding iodine concentrations of nonionic CM, it is not surprising that they are more neurotoxic.

It has been shown that the BBB may take between 5 min and 3 h to be reconstituted after a carotid infusion of hypertonic solutions, depending on the condition of the infusion [6] and so repeated injections of ionic CM within several minutes of each other may increase the risk of neurotoxic effects. Sodium salts of ionic CM have been shown to be more neurotoxic than equivalent concentrations of meglumine/methylglucamine salts. Once having crossed the BBB, neurotoxicity of an ionic CM is therefore due to its chemotoxic effect, which is related to its molecular structure, rather than to an osmotic effect [6].

A number of substances have been studied to see if they have a protective role against potential neurotoxicity of CM. Experimentally, both low molecular weight dextran and steroids have been shown to have protective effects [8], but their routine use has not been justified clinically.

In general, although the above effects on the BBB may occur during neuroangiography, particularly with hypertonic ionic CM, most neurological deficits associated with neuroangiography are probably related to ischaemic complications of catheter technique rather than the result of the toxic effects of the CM [3, 6]. On the other hand, the seizures that have been reported in 0.2% of cerebral angiograms and 0.4% of arch aortograms [3] are probably related to the CM crossing the BBB because of pre-existing pathology or osmotic breakdown.

Transient cortical blindness occasionally occurs during or following an uncomplicated vertebral angiogram, and this complication may be a direct effect of the CM on the occipital lobe. Patients with ischaemic cerebrovascular disease or subarachnoid haemorrhage have a great incidence of neurological complications from neuroangiography [3, 6]. This may be related to an increased risk of arterial embolism or haemodynamic effects such as spasm, but there may be greater sensitivity to the CM itself, perhaps due to increased BBB permeability [6].

Spinal cord injury as a result of uncomplicated aortography or, more specifically, spinal angiography, is well recognized and, although such injury may be the result of catheter technique, many feel that permanent spinal cord injury may be due to the direct neurotoxic effect of the CM [3].

Intrathecal Contrast Media

The interface between the CSF and the brain is at the pia mater overlying the brain surface and the ependyma lining the ventricular system. Unlike the physiological barrier of the BBB between the blood and brain parenchyma, there appears to be no barrier between the CSF and the extracellular fluid of the brain [5, 6], and water-soluble molecules such as CM appear to enter the brain parenchyma by simple diffusion into the extracellular space. Brain penetration by water-soluble CM after intrathecal injection has been well documented experimentally [5, 6] and clinically [5] and so therefore such CM comes into direct contact with the neuronal cells. Such penetration occurs with both ionic and nonionic CM to a similar degree.

Intrathecal nonionic CM have been shown to cause electroencephalographic (EEG) changes, presumably due to this brain penetration, and such changes appear to result from the chemotoxic rather than the osmotic action of the CM [5, 6]. Seizures have been reported [6] even with the latest nonionic CM and therefore a history of seizures or medication known to reduce the seizure threshold are relative contraindications to intrathecal CM.

Neuropsychological reactions such as behavioural disturbances, confusion, amnesia, agitation and hallucinations have been reported after intrathecal nonionic CM [5, 6], a frequency of 13%–38% being reported with metrizamide, and they have not been completely eliminated with the later nonionic CM. Such reactions are presumably due to the passage of the intrathecal CM into the extracellular fluid of the brain.

Headache frequently follows the injection of intrathecal CM. An incidence of 38% has been reported [7], the highest frequency following cervical myelography with lumbar puncture and the lowest frequency occurring with a C1–2 puncture [7]. Overall, leakage of CSF following thecal puncture is probably the most important factor in provoking headache, not CM toxicity, as the frequency of headache after myelography using lumbar puncture has been reported as approximately the same as that following diagnostic lumbar puncture [7].

Adhesive arachnoiditis has been reported following lumbar myelography using ionic water-soluble CM [7], but this does not appear to be a problem with the latest generation of nonionic CM.

There is a continuing debate regarding the efficacy of epidural and intrathecal steroids and their possible promotion of arachnoiditis. Therefore, for medico-legal reasons alone, the injection of intraspinal steroids is currently inadvisable.

References

1. Bradbury MW (1988) Transport across the blood-brain barrier. In: Neuwelt EA (ed) Implications of the blood-brain barrier and its manipulation. Plenum, New York, pp 119–134
2. Hilal SK (1966) Haemodynamic responses in the cerebral vessels to angiographic contrast media. Acta Radiol 5:211–231
3. Junck J, Marshall WH (1983) Neurotoxicity of radiological contrast agents. Ann Neurol 13:469–484
4. Murphy DJ (1973) Cerebrovascular permeability after meglumine iothalamate administration. Neurology 23:926–936
5. Sage MR (1983) Kinetics of water-soluble contrast media in the central nervous system. AJNR 4:897–906
6. Sage MR (1989) Neuroangiography. In: Skucas J (ed) Radiographic contrast agents, 2nd edn. Aspen, Rockville, pp 170–188
7. Skalpe IO, Nakstad P (1988) Myelography with iohexol (omnipaque): a clinical report with special reference to the adverse effects. Neuroradiology 30:169–174
8. Sovak M (1984) Contrast media for imaging of the central nervous system. In: Sovak M (ed) Radio Contrast Agents. Springer, Berlin Heidelberg New York, pp 295–340 (Handbook of experimental pharmacology, vol 73)

3.11 Do Contrast Media Affect Blood Vessel Walls?

F. Laerum

It is generally accepted that hyperosmolar ionic CM may cause peripheral artery injection pain and may have neurotoxic effects after cerebral angiography or engender deep venous thrombosis and phlebitis following phlebography. Over the years, various in vitro and in vivo models have been employed to demonstrate that such effects are often due to vessel wall injury. Damage to the intima caused by CM exposure has been demonstrated by several authors by means of silver staining of the vascular endothelium of aorta or vena cava in rats. Activation of coagulation factors by underlying tissue after denuding subendothelial structures may then cause thrombosis. Grabowski [4] employed a microvessel system and found that, at a concentration of CM in culture medium of 20% by volume, monolayer endothelial cell morphology was less altered by the nonionic low-osmolar CM iohexol than by the ionic CM diatrizoate or ioxaglate and that monolayer production of prostacyclin was enhanced by the low-osmolar ioxaglate compared to saline controls.

Schneider et al. examined the effects of diatrizoate, iohexol and ioxilan on the endothelium of rabbit aortic rings and on endothelial-derived relaxing factor (dilator response) [14]. Hyperosmolar diatrizoate produced intercellular gaps and vesicles containing myelin figures as seen on electron microscopy and after 15 minutes of incubation, the dilator response was irreversibly reduced to 49%. In contrast, iohexol and ioxilan produced just some irregularities in cell and vesicle borders, and the contact time for iohexol had to be raised to 60 min to produce a dilator response similar to that with diatrizoate, even after this period; the similarly nonionic low-osmolar CM ioxilan still did not produce such a response.

The role of CM in addition to effects of manipulation of catheters, guidewires and other intravascular devices or pharmaceuticals remains to be clarified. Occlusions or reocclusions of arterial stenoses or recanalized segmental obstructions may be seen in connection with angioplasty. In such cases, injury to the vessel wall by mechanical manipulation of catheters or guidewires may also be involved.

In the veins, there is clear evidence of deep venous thrombosis in the lower limbs following phlebography with hyperosmolar CM. The reported incidence varies from 6%–26%, probably due to differences in contact time, CM volume and wash-out procedures. This iatrogenic problem may be avoided by using low-osmolar compounds. Lowering the CM concentration or prophylactic anticoagulant treatment may also decrease the incidence. Studies on venous endothelium in vivo and in vitro have revealed injurious effects of hyperosmolar CM. We performed a lethality test on human endothelial cells in culture. The cells were derived from umbilical cord veins. When the cell cultures were in confluence, they were labelled with ^{51}Cr and then exposed to various CM and concentrations for 10 min or 24 h.

The 10-min exposure was performed with ordinary 300 mg I/ml contrast media solutions added to the cell cultures after removal of the cell culture medium. This model should mimic the local effects of a pulsed CM injection into a small vein. The ^{51}Cr release from these cultures was up to six times higher following exposure to hyperosmolar

CM (diatrizoate, metrizoate) than to the least toxic agent, iopamidol. The other low-osmolar CM tested (ioxaglate, metrizamide, iohexol) had about the same effects as 0.9% saline.

In the 24-h test, the CM were added in decreasing concentrations of 21.3–2.1 vol% to the cell culture medium, thus testing general biocompatibility of the agents. The cell toxicity was (in decreasing order): diatrizoate, metrizoate, ioxaglate, iopamidol, metrizamide, iohexol. Diatrizoate led to 99% cell death in this model, iohexol 40% at the same concentration. The strongest osmolality-independent toxic effect was caused by the dimeric CM ioxaglate. In both the designs, the results revealed significant differences among the various CM as to endothelial damage. Hyperosmolality was the most important noxious factor, but we also noted that ionic CM had more chemotoxic effects than nonionic CM media, apart from osmolality. Thiesen and Muetzel infused CM or sorbitol for 2 min into mesenteric veins of rabbits [15]: they concluded that hyperosmolarity is the causal factor in endothelial damage, since electron microscopy revealed shrinkage of cell cytoplasm and in nuclear material. Inflammatory processes in the venous wall may also be enhanced by the exposure to contrast media [13].

In conclusion, CM may damage the vessel wall, in particular the endothelium. The injury is primarily linked to the CM osmolality, but chemotoxicity also plays a role. Low-osmolar CM are better and the nonionic solutions seem preferable to the ionic.

References

1. Albrechtsson U, Olsson C-G (1979) Thrombosis after phlebography: a comparison of two contrast media. Cardiovasc Radiol 2:9–14
2. Bettmann MA, Salzman EW, Rosenthal D et al (1980) Reduction of venous thrombosis complicating phlebography. AJR 134:1169–1172
3. Bromann T, Olsson O (1949) Experimental study of contrast media for cerebral angiography with reference to possible injurious effects on the cerebral blood vessels. Acta Radiol 31:321–334
4. Grabowski EF (1989) Effects of contrast media on endothelial cell monolayers under controlled flow conditions. In: Enge I, Edgren P (eds) Patient safety and adverse events in contrast medium examinations. No. 816 Elsevier/Excerpta Medica, Amsterdam, pp 85–95 (International ongress series, no 816)
5. Hol R, Skjerven O (1954) Spinal cord damage in abdominal angiography. Acta Radiol 42:276–284
6. Hörup A, Eliassen B, Reimer-Jensen A, Praestholm J (1982) Comparison of Hexabrix and Urografin in the study of post-phlebographic thrombotic side effects. In: Amiél M (ed) Contrast media in Radiology. Springer, Berlin Heidelberg New York, pp 231–232
7. Laerum F (1987) Cytotoxic effects of six angiographic contrast media on human endothelium in culture. Acta Radiol 28:99–105
8. Laerum F (1983) Acute damage to human endothelial cells by brief exposure to contrast media in vitro. Radiology 147:681–684
9. Laerum F, Holm HA (1981) Postphlebographic thrombosis. A double blind study with methylglucamine metrizoate and metrizamide. Radiology 140:651–654
10. Mersereau WA, Robertson HR (1961) Observations on venous endothelial injury following the injection of various radiographic contrast media in the rat. J Neurosurg 18:289–294
11. Nyman U, Almén T (1980) Effects of contrast media on aortic endothelium. Experiments in the rat with non-ionic

monomeric and mono-acidic dimeric contrast media. Acta Radiol Suppl 362:65–71

12. Raininko R (1979) Role of hypertonicity in the endothelial injury caused by angiographic contrast media. Acta Radiol 20:410–416

13. Ritchie WGM, Lynch PR, Stewart GJ (1974) The effect of contrast media on normal and inflamed canine veins. Invest Radiol 9:444–455

14. Schneider KM, Ham KN, Friedhuber A, Rand MJ (1988) Functional and morphologic effects of ioxilan, iohexol and diatrizoate on endothelial cells. Invest Radiol 23 (Suppl 1):S147–149

15. Thiesen B, Muetzel W (1990) Effects of contrast media on venous endothelium of rabbits. Invest Radiol 25:121–126

16. Zinner G, Gottlob R (1959) Die gefäßschädigende Wirkung verschiedener Röntgenkontrastmittel, vergleichende Untersuchungen. Fortschr Roentgenstr 91:507–511

CHAPTER 4

Determination of Risk Factors Regarding the Administration of Contrast Media

4.1 What Are the Known Risks of Contrast Media Use?

W. Clauß

In prospective clinical studies involving great numbers of cases, nonionic, low-osmolar CM proved to be much better tolerated than their ionic, hyperosmolar counterparts. This holds, above all, for the rates of mild to moderately severe side effects. However, these favorable results for nonionic CM also clearly hold for the rate of severe reactions and for examinations involving at risk patients (Table 4.1.1).

Even though the number and intensity of almost every adverse reaction (ADR) is reduced when nonionic CM are administered, previous wide-ranging experience has shown that the general risks and profile of side effects still remain.

Even in the presence of all of the main risks in the following list, nonionic X-ray CM can still be used in conjunction with concomitant pro-

Table 4.1.1. Adverse reactions after intravenous injection of ionic and nonionic contrast media

Reference	No. of patients		Adverse Reaction Rate (%)					
			Total		Severe reactions		Risk patients only	
	Ionic	Nonionic	Ionic	Nonionic	Ionic	Nonionic	Ionic	Nonionic
Schrott et al. 1986	–	50 642	–	2.1	–	0.01	–	4.1 (History of CM ADR)
								3.3 (History of allergy)
Palmer 1988	79 278	30 268	3.8	1.2	0.10	0.01	10.3	1.3 (Different risks)
Wolf 1989	6 006	7 170	4.1	0.7	0.4	0.0	–	–
Katayama et al. 1990	169 284	168 363	12.7	3.1	0.22	0.04	44.7	11.2 (History of CM ARD)
							23.9	6.9 (History of allergy)

ADR, adverse reactions; CM, contrast media

phylactic measures, if strictly indicated. This presupposes, however, that the examining physician estimates the risks involved by taking a careful case history, is aware of any known pathogenetic interrelationships, takes prophylactic measures and prescribes a follow-up examination if necessary.

Risks that can result in an increased rate of side effects or further deterioration of organ function include:
- Hypersensitivity to CM
- Allergies
- Manifest and latent hyperthyroidism
- Bland nodular goitre
- Severe cardiovascular insufficiency
- Respiratory disorder
- Renal insufficiency
- Diabetes mellitus
- Paraproteinaemia
- Phaeochromocytoma
- Dehydration
- Autoimmune disorders
- Sickle-cell anaemia
- Patients over the age of 60

References

1. Katayama H, Yamaguchi K, Kozuka T, Takashima T, Seez P, Matsuura K (1990) Adverse reactions to ionic and non-ionic contrast media. Radiology 175:621–628
2. Palmer FJ (1989) The RACR survey of intravenous contrast media reactions. Australas Radiol 32:426–428
3. Schrott KM, Behrends B, Clauß W, Kaufmann J, Lehnert J (1986) Iohexol in der Ausscheidungsurographie. Fortschr. Med. 7:153–156
4. Wolf GL, Arenson RL, Cross AP (1989) A prospective trial of ionic versus non-ionic contrast agents in routine clinical practice. AJR 152:939–944

4.2 Does Known X-Ray Contrast Media Hypersensitivity and a History of Allergies Mean Increased Risk in Examinations Using X-Rays Contrast Media?

W. Clauß

X-ray CM (as well as local and intravenous anaesthetics and colloidal volume substitutes) can lead to pseudoallergic reactions. In clinical terms, the latter may resemble classic, IgE-mediated anaphylaxis, but are rarely of immunological origin. For this reason, they are termed pseudoanaphylactic. The pathomechanism upon which they are based is still unknown, but possible explanations include: complement activation, the direct release of mediators, such as histamine and serotonin, interactions with the coagulation, fibrinolytic and kallikrein-kinin systems and the involvement of neuropsychogenic reflexes.

As the large-scale statistical survey by Katayama [2] demonstrated, the side-effect rate can be decreased by roughly a factor of four by intravenously administering nonionic X-ray CM (3.1%) instead of ionic X-ray CM (12.7%).

For a group of patients with known histories of hypersensitive reactions to the X-ray CM being used, the risk of the occurrence of renewed side effects in an examination in which X-ray CM are once again administered is roughly five times greater than the risk for a previously reaction-free group (with nonionic

X-ray CM from 2.2% to 11.3% and with ionic, hyperosmolar X-ray CM from 9.0% to 44.0%).

Patients with histories of allergy also demonstrate increased risk when X-ray CM are administered. In the Katayama study, the side-effect rate rose by roughly a factor of 2.5 or 2, when one moved from the nonallergy to the allergy group (in intravenous administration of nonionic X-ray CM, moving from 2.8% to 6.9% and of ionic X-ray CM from 11.7% to 23.4%).

Further studies of large numbers of patients confirmed Katayama's results [1, 3–5] and attest to the clearly lower potential possessed by nonionic as opposed to ionic X-ray for triggering pseudoanaphylaxis. However, a residual risk still exists and has to be further reduced by means of suitable prophylactic measures, especially for patients with defined risks.

Anaphylactoid reactions occurs more frequently after intravenous than after intraarterial administration (release of mediators from the pulmonary mast cells increased by high concentrations of CM). Though it is very rare, such a reaction cannot be ruled out following the intracavitary administration of X-ray CM.

References

1. Gerstmann BB (1991) Epidemiologic critique of the report on adverse reactions to ionic and nonionic media by the Japanese Committee on the Safety of Contrast Media. Radiology 178:787
2. Katayama H, Yamaguchi K, Kozuka T, Takashima T, Seez P, Matsuura K (1990) Adverse reactions to ionic and nonionic contrast media. Radiology: 175:621–628
3. Palmer FJ (1988) The RACR survey of intravenous contrast media reactions – final report. Australas Radiol 4
4. Schrott KM, Behrends B, Clauß W, Kaufmann J, Lehnert J (1986) IOHE-XOL in der Ausscheidungsurographie: Ergebnisse des Drug-monitorings. Fortschr Med 7:153/51–156/54
5. Wolf GL, Arenson RL, Cross AP (1989) A prospective trial of ionic vs. nonionic contrast agents in routine clinical practice: comparison of adverse effects. AJR 152:939

4.3 Does an Existing Iodine Allergy Mean Increased Risk in Examinations Using X-Ray Contrast Media?

W. Clauß

An iodine allergy is a type-IV contact dermatitis reaction. Thus, intravasculary administered X-ray CM do not necessarily lead to pseudoanaphylaxis in iodine allergy. The occurrence of haematogenous contact dermatitis cannot, however, be ruled out, since X-ray CM do contain a very small percentage of iodine as an impurity [1].

References

1. Ring J (1988) Pseudoallergische Arzneimittel-Reaktionen. Angewandte Allergologie, 2. Aufl., MMV Medizin, München, 223–234

4.4 Why Does the Administration of Iodinated Contrast Media to Patients with Manifest or Latent Hyperthyroidism Represent a Risk?

B. Glöbel

Hyperfunction of the thyroid gland only leads to a hyperthyroid metabolic condition if the thyroid has enough iodide at its disposal to be able to produce excessive amounts of iodinated thyroid hormones. In a geographical area of iodine deficiency, (e.g. Germany), cases of hyperthyroidism only then appear if the quantity of iodide supplied is increased. This occurs, for example, in the administration of iodinated X-ray CM. Here, a possible exacerbation of the symptoms of hyperthyroidism can occur with the real risk of lapse into a thyrotoxic crisis. For this reason, hyperthyroidism should be treated and under control prior to an examination of such patients with iodinated X-ray CM. Emergency cases of untreated hyperthyroidism or autonomy of the thyroid gland can be treated with thyroid depressants. However, a physician experienced in the diagnosis and therapy of diseases of the thyroid gland should be consulted as soon as possible after the CM examination. The period of intensive observation of the patient should run at least 8 weeks. The following table provides an introductory guide to the dosage of antithyroid agents (Table 4.4.1).

Table 4.4.1. Comparative dosing of thyroid depressants in relation to carbimazole 1

Generic name	Carbimazole	Methimazole Thiamozol	Propylthiouracil (PTU)	Perchlorate
Chemic term	3-methyl-2-thioxo-4-imidazoline-1-carbon dioxide-ethylester	1-methyl-2-mer-captoimidazole	4-propyl-2-thiouracil	Sodium perchlorate Potassium perchlorate
Commercial preparations	Carbimazol 10 mg "Henning" Neo-Morphazole Neo-Thyreostat	Favistan	Propycil Thyreostat II	Irenat
Comparable doses	1	1 1/2	ca. 8–12	19
Initial doses, month 1	15–80 mg/day	60–120 mg/day	150–600 mg/day	600-1200 mg/day (week 1)
Subsequent doses, month 2	5–15 mg/day	5–20 mg/day	25–100 mg/day	150–300 mg/day (weeks 2–8)

4.5 Why Does the Administration of Iodinated Contrast Media Represent a Risk to Patients with Bland Nodular Goitre?

B. Glöbel

Almost all bland nodular goitres are the result of a longer-term iodine deficiency. In iodine deficiency, the thyroid is constantly stimulated via the regulatory organs of the hypothalamus and the pituitary gland to absorb more iodine and to produce more thyroid hormone. It appears that in this situation autonomous thyroid cells increasingly arise that are no longer subject to regulation. If such patients are suddenly supplied with an increased amount of iodide, there is a danger that the autonomous thyroid regions will produce too much thyroid hormone and thereby create a hyperthyroid metabolic condition.

The hyperthyroid metabolic condition is limited by the excretion of the additional iodide. The amount of iodide supplied by more modern iodinated X-ray CM is usually only sufficient to temporarily remedy the existing iodine deficiency.

Considerations for Diagnostically Necessary Examinations with Iodinated X-Ray Contrast Media

A hyperthyroid metabolic condition is most likely to be triggered in newborns and small children because of the relatively small volume of distribution. High iodide concentrations in the plasma can result, which in turn leads to an inhibition of thyroid hormone synthesis. Transient hypothyroidism is involved here, which as a rule does not last longer than 4 days. As a precautionary measure, a test of thyroid function can be performed after ca. 8 days. Should a hypothyroid metabolic condition still exist at this time, then thyroid hormone substitution therapy can be implemented. The risk to newborns following the examination of their mothers with iodinated X-ray CM should be clinically insignificant. The passage of iodide into the mother's milk ranges from a few percent to a maximum of ten percent. The second group at risk through the increased supply of iodide is represented by those patients known to have latent or manifest hyperthyroidism. In these patients, for different reasons, autonomous tissue sections exist in the thyroid that increase production of thyroid hormones when the supply of iodide is increased. Here, too, transient hyperthyroidism is involved in most cases; after excretion of the iodide supplied, it recedes and does not require treatment.

The risk of a thyrotoxic crisis cannot presently be predicted with certainty. In Germany it can be assumed that this risk is at maximum $1:50,000$. It is probably much smaller since the more recent iodinated X-ray CM used intravenously are extremely biologically stable and are only contaminated with small amounts of free iodide in production. The additional amount of iodide supplied ranges as a rule between 0.1 and 10 mg per examination. Such amounts of iodide are felt

to be completely acceptable in iodized salt and they are, for example,
much smaller than are contained in
the so-called 'iodine' tablets that are
recommended for use in the reduction of internal radiation exposure
after nuclear catastrophes.

4.6 Does Underlying Cardiovascular Disease Constitute an Increased Risk in Contrast Media Administration?

P. Dawson

Severe Cardiovascular insufficiency

CM are able to produce marked peripheral vasodilatation with a sometimes profound fall in systemic
blood pressure [1]. Patients with
normal cardiac function can raise a
reflex tachycardia without difficulty,
patients with poor cardiac reserve,
however, may undergo what
amounts to a cardiac function stress
test on administration of a contrast
agent and may be at risk. Attacks of
angina are not infrequently observed
in patients with ischaemic heart disease undergoing contrast examinations. CM injected directly into the
coronary arteries actually may increase coronary blood flow for a
short time but this appears to occur
only in areas of relatively normal
vascularity and not in areas of abnormal vascularity [1]. There appears, as a consequence, to be a
steal phenomenon which renders
ischaemic areas even more ischaemic and the effect is entirely unde-

sirable. Patients with ischaemic
heart disease are therefore at risk in
this regard. Intracoronary and left
ventricular contrast agents also have
adverse effects on pump function
and on cardiac electrophysiology [1].
In patients with pre-existing ischaemic heart disease the effects may be
more marked and more prolonged
with a greater propensity to ventricular fibrillation [3].

As regards peripheral injection of
contrast agents, as in intravenous
urography and CT enhancement, it
may be possible to exaggerate the
importance of cardiac disease. Katayama [2] in his recent large-scale
study of adverse effects of ionic and
nonionic CM did not observe any
significantly increased risk of problems in the older age groups as
would be expected on the basis of an
anticipated increasing incidence of
cardiac disease in an aging population.

References

1. Dawson P (1989) Cardiovascular effects of contrast agents. Am J Cardiol 64:2E–9E
2. Katayama H et al. (1990) Adverse reactions to ionic and non-ionic contrast media. A report from the Japanese Committee on the Safety of Contrast Media. Radiology 175:621–628
3. Wolf GL, Kraft L, Kilzer K (1978) Contrast agents lower ventricular fibrillation threshold. Radiology 129:215–217

4.7 Why Is Pre-existing Lung Disease a Risk for the Administration of Contrast Media?

P. Dawson

As discussed elsewhere, CM administered directly into the bronchopulmonary tree or into the lymphatics or peripheral veins are capable of producing a number of adverse effects in the lungs, including an increase in interstitial pulmonary water [2] with impairment of both compliance and diffusion [1], the production of a routine subclinical bronchospasm and an occasional more dramatic bronchospasm. Patients with pre-existing lung function disturbances may therefore be at increased risk. These include those with already impaired compliance and diffusion and those with a tendency to bronchospasm, not only asthmatics, but also those with chronic obstructive airways disease with an element of bronchospasm.

References

1. Dawson P, Pitfield J, Britton J (1983) Contrast media and bronchospasm: a study with iopamidol. Clin Radiol 34:227–230
2. Slutsky RA, Mackney DB, Peck WN, Higgins CB (1983) Extravascular lung water: effects of ionic and non-ionic contrast media. Radiology 149:375–381

4.8 Why Is Pre-existing Renal Impairment a Risk in the Administration of Contrast Media?

J. E. Scherberich

The more serious the pre-existing renal insufficiency, the greater the risk that the further reduction in renal function induced by CM will not remain temporary and asymptomatic. Acute renal failure can result. The first clinical signs are polyuria or oligoanuria and, in roentgenological terms, a persistent nephrogram. The following symptoms are observed in succession: oedema formation, increase in weight, fatigue, dyspnoea caused by pulmonary oedema, possible hyperventilation, presternal pains, muscular weakness, fasciculation, pruritus, tendency to bleed, convulsions and coma.

In pathogenetic terms, there are various possible mechanisms of CM-related nephrotoxicity that can trigger acute kidney failure. Understandably, their effects on an already functionally impaird kidney are usually much more serious than on a healthy organ.

4.9 Why Is Pre-existing Diabetes Mellitus a Risk in the Administration of Contrast Media?

J. E. Scherberich

In diabetic nephropathy, especially in patients with juvenile diabetes and insulin-dependent diabetes mellitus, or in these inadequately prepared for CM administration, there is a very high risk of CM-induced conditions ranging from the serious deterioration of kidney function to acute kidney failure.

Pathological changes such as diabetic nephropathy with glomerular sclerosis and tubulointerstitial metaplasia do not usually occur in diabetes mellitus until after more than 10 years in half of the patients. So until then diabetes mellitus does not represent an increased clinical risk for the administration of CM.

In order to estimate the clinical risk profile in patients with diabetes mellitus, at least the current serum creatinine concentration should be known (along with blood pressure and initial weight) before CM is administered.

with subsequent kidney failure. The results of in vivo investigations did not support this hypothesis, though. More recent retrospective studies on patients with multiple myeloma did not indicate any CM-influenced change in renal excretion, even in cases of pre-existing renal insufficiency. In accordance with these results, the diagnosis of plasmacytoma/myeloma is today no longer regarded as an absolute contraindication to CM-enhanced X-ray examinations. However, the use of nonionic CM and the adequate hydration of the patient prior to examination (1000–1500 ml 0.9% NaCl solution) are strongly recommended. The CM doses should also be kept as low as possible and all potentially nephrotoxic medications discontinued prior to examination.

4.10 Why Is Pre-existing Paraproteinaemia a Risk in the Administration of Contrast Media?

J. E. Scherberich

Until a few years ago, the occasional in vitro observation of the aggregation of CM with alkaline Bence Jones proteins or the high-molecular-weight Tamm-Horsfall uromucoid was used to explain the isolated cases of acute kidney failure previously observed in myeloma patients following urography. The precipitated paraprotein was supposed to have led to obstructive nephropathy (acute "cast nephropathy")

4.11 How Can the Risk of Provoking a Hypertensive Crisis in Patients with Phaeochromocytoma Be Reduced?

P. Dawson

Evidence that intravascular CM may be associated with hypertensive crises in patients with phaeochromocytoma is anecdotal and no large studies have been performed. Small series with a proportion of hypertensive responses have been observed in arteriography [1], in adrenal phlebography [3] and in enhanced CT [5] in patients with these tumours. In so far as the phenomenon is documented, α-adrenergic blockade appears to be helpful in preventing a life-threatening crisis. However, occasional deaths ascribed to the phenomenon have been reported even relatively recently [4]. No evidence is available concerning the status of low osmolality agents, ionic or nonionic, in this regard. Only the argument from first principles may be called in aid, namely that nonionic CM are more biocompatible in general terms and it seems reasonable to use these agents in such patients.

Dawson has suggested a possible mechanism [2]. The cells of the adrenal medulla are histologically closely related to autonomic ganglion cells and are innervated by preganglionic sympathetic fibres. Stimulation of these fibres raises blood pressure by release of adrenalin and noradrenalin into the circulation. Before the rise of blood pressure there is sometimes a fall which is increased after administration of physostigmine and abolished by atropine – evidence that acetylcholine as first liberated at stimulated nerve endings is the transmitter involved. Indeed, acetylcholine has been identified in the adrenal vein following sympathetic stimulation. Perhaps the mechanisms involved are, therefore, cholinergic.

Prophylaxis consists of adequate α-adrenergic blockade and the drug of choice was phentolamine, but some authorities prefer combined α and β blockade because phaeochromocytomas secrete both adrenaline and noradrenaline (and other mediators). This may be achieved by a labetalol infusion during the procedure titrated against the blood pressure.
Hypertensive crises, if they nevertheless occur, may be treated with intravenous phentolamine, 5–10 mg, with 0.5 mg/min infusion if required. The effect is rapid and short-lived.

References

1. Christenson R, Smith CW, Burko M (1976) Arteriographic manifestation of phaeochromacytoma. AJR 126:567–575
2. Dawson P (1987) Cholinergic mechanisms in contrast media induced adverse reactions. In: Parvez Z, Moncada S, Sorak M (eds) Contrast media: biologic effects and clinical application. CRC Press, Boca Raton
3. Fisch HP, Reutter FW (1976) Paralytic ileus in phaeochromocytoma. Possible correlation with an attempt at adrenal phlebography. Schweiz Med Wochenschr 106:1187–1191
4. Kashimura S, Umetsu K, Suzuki T (1979) A sudden death from phaeochromocytoma following arteriography. Jpn Legal Med 33:7–12
5. Raisanen J, Shapiro B, Glazer GM (1984) Plasma catacholamines in phaeochromocytoma: effect of urographic contrast media. AJR 143:43–46

4.12 Can Dehydration Before Contrast Media Administration Be Recommended Today?

J. E. Scherberich

Dehydration

All of the CM available today (except for IOTROLAN and IODIXANOL) are more or less osmotically active substances and absorb water from their environment. For this reason, patients in dehydrated states should be adequately hydrated with up to 2000 ml 0.9 NaCl solution prior to CM administration. Electrolyte loss must also be compensated for. Going without liquids for 12 h and more, previously recommended for the most concentrated CM excretion possible and a resulting improved demonstration of pyelogram and ureters, is considered obsolete today for reasons of increased risk of nephrotoxicity and because better tolerated CM can now be administered in higher doses to yield to diagnostically satisfactory X-rays without water deprivation.

In isolated cases where it is necessary to extend the examination and administer high doses of hyperosmolar, CM (= > 300 ml), water and electrolytes need to be supplemented.

4.13 Are Patients with Autoimmune Disorders at Any Particular Risk on Contrast Media Administration?

P. Dawson

There have been a number of case reports over the last decade of adverse reactions to a variety of iodinated CM in patients known to be suffering from autoimmune disorders [1–6]. It is always difficult to be certain about cause and effect and patients with such disorders may have exacerbations of their symptoms from time to time. However, the exceptionally dramatic episodes and florid symptomatology displayed by some of those patients shortly following administration of CM suggests the possibility of a link.

Some cases involved a nonionic agent, others an ionic agent. Variously, intra-arterial, intravenous and intrathecal routes of administration were involved. If the circumstantial evidence of a link is accepted, we might speculate that the ability of CM to activate complement might be involved in the aetiology.

Caution is indicated. As always the need for a contrast examination in those patients should be carefully assessed and alternatives considered. If a decision is made to perform the contrast examination, it is suggested on purely empirical grounds that corticosteroid prophylaxis for 24–48 h before the examination be used.

References

1. Gelmers HJ (1984) Exacerbation of systemic lupus erythematosus, aseptic meningitis and acute mental symptoms, following metrizamide lumbar myelography. Neuroradiology 26:–65–66
2. Goodfellow T et al (1986) Fatal acute vasculitis after high-dose urography with iohexol. Br J Radiol 59:620–621
3. Kaur JS et al (1982) Acute renal failure following arteriography in a patient with polyarteritis nodosa. JAMA 6:833–834
4. Reuter FW, Eugster C (1985) Akuter Jodismus mit Sialadenitis, allergischer Vaskulitis und Konjunktivitis nach Verabreichung iodhaltiger Kontrastmittel. Schweiz Med Wochenschr 115:1646–1651
5. Savill JS et al (1988) Fatal Stevens-Johnson syndrome following urography with iopamidol in systemic lupus erythematosus. Postgrad Med J 64:392–394
6. Vaillant L et al (1990) Iododerma and acute respiratory distress with leucocytoclastic vasculitis following the intravenous injection of contrast medium. Clin Dermat 15:232–233

4.14 Does the Administration of Iodinated Contrast Media to Patients with Sickle Cell Anaemia Result in Further Change in Erythrocytic Shape?

R. Dickerhoff

Sickle cell anaemia is an inherited disease in which an abnormal haemoglobin, haemoglobin S (HbS), is formed. HbS exhibits the property of precipitating into long, rigid forms (not only in deoxygenated conditions but in hypertonic media as well) and of forcing a sickle-shape upon the cell. Sickle cells in the blood have shortened longevity and there is chronic haemolytic anaemia and, because of increased viscosity, may be vascular occlusions [6].

The sickle-cell mutation arose in Africa and spread to the Mediterranean region via commercial routes and to the New World via the slave trade. In the last 30 years, sickle cell anaemia has also become frequent in northern Europe through the influx of immigrants, above all from the Mediterranean countries and Africa [3].

In 10%–15% of all sickle-cell patients, cerebral infarcts occur, which in some cases make arteriography necessary [7]. Conventional, ionic CM with their high osmolality (0.9–2.5 osm/kg H_2O) lead to increased sickling [2, 8] in sickle-cell blood in vitro; this results from the water loss they cause in the erythrocytes and the resulting higher concentration of HbS (a rise in mean corpuscular haemoglobin concentration, MCHC).

Since Richards and Nulsen [8] reported on two sickle-cell patients with severe neurological damage following carotid angiography, it has been recommended that prior to every arteriography HbS levels be reduced below 20% by means of a partial exchange transfusion in order to prevent intravascular sicking [4, 5, 10]. On the other hand, intravenous pyelography can be performed without prior exchange transfusion. The more recently developed, nonionic CM (0.4–0.8 osm/kg H_2O) lead in vitro to much less sickling and to a lesser increase in MCHC [9]. In vivo examinations are presently being carried out in London for the first time (M. Brosovic, personal communication). In cerebral and pulmonary arteriography, it is still advisable to perform a partial exchange transfusion prior to CM administration in order to avoid stimulation of an occlusion due to intermittently sickling cells in the vessels. These "ephemeral occlusions" are no longer found after an exchange transfusion; only genuine vascular occlusions remain. CM are administered to sickle-cell patients in normal doses.

References

1. Cheatham MI, Brackett CE (1965) Problems in management of subarachnoid hemorrhage in sickle cell anemia. J Neurosurg 23:488–493
2. Dickerhoff R, Schwalber I, Bode U, Kohne E, Kleihauer E (1990) Sichelzellerkrankungen in West-Deutschland. Dtsch Ärztebl 87:1466–1471
3. Gerald B, Sebes JL, Langston JW (1980) Cerebral infarction secondary to

sickle cell disease: arteriographic findings. AJR 134:1209–1212

4. Olivieri Russell M, Goldberg HI, Reiss L et al (1976) Transfusion therapy for cerebrovascular abnormalities in sickle cell disease. J Pediatr 88:382–387
5. Powars DR (1975) The natural history of sickle cell disease – the first 10 years. Semin Hematol 12:267–285
6. Portnoy BA, Herion JC (1972) Neurological manifestations in sickle cell disease. Ann Int Med 76:643–652
7. Rao VM, Rao AK, Steiner RM et al (1982) The effect of ionic and nonionic contrast media on the sickling phenomenon. Radiology 144:291–293
8. Richards D, Nulsen FE (1971) Angiographic media and the sickling phenomenon. Surg Forum 22:403–404
9. Sarnaik S, Soorya D, Kim J, Ravindranath Y, Lusher J (1979) Periodic transfusions for sickle cell anemia and CNS infarction. Am J Dis Child 133:1254–1257

4.15 Are Contrast Media-Induced Side Effects Dependent on Age?

H. Katayama

Among several risk factors for CM reactions, the age of the patient is thought to be one of the principal ones. As far as overall reactions are concerned, Shehadi reported that they were more prevalent in the third and fourth decades. Incidence was lowest at either end of the age spectrum [5, 7]. According to Ansell [2], the incidence rates of minor reactions were highest in the 20- to 29-year age group and tended to be lower in younger and older patients. Intermediate reactions showed a similar trend. The severe reactions showed a more uniform distribution, with perhaps a slight predominance in the older age group. These data are based on patients administered conventional high osmolar ionic CM.

Katayama [3] has reported on a large survey of adverse reactions to ionic and nonionic CM. It showed the highest incidence of overall reactions in the third and fourth decades. There was no definite trend for severe reactions but with a slight predominance in the third to fifth decade. This was true both with ionic and nonionic CM though with an indistinct trend in severe reactions with nonionic CM (Table 4.15.1). Parameters estimated for the selected logistic regression model for severe adverse reactions show the odds ratios to be: under 9 years 0.58; 10–49 years 1.0; and over 50 years 0.68 [4]. As far as fatal reactions were concerned, Shehadi reported that the peak incidence of fatal reactions was observed in the sixth to seventh decade [6]. The cause of death is thought to be mainly due to cardiovascular collapse secondary to administration of high osmolar CM. Ansell's [1] results agreed with this trend.

In conclusion, overall adverse reactions are commoner in the early middle age group. Fatal reactions are throught to be commoner in the group over 50 years of age.

References

1. Ansell G et al (1980) The current status of reactions to i. v. CM. Invest Radiol [Suppl]: 32–39
2. Ansell G (1970) Adverse reactions to CA. Invest Radiol 6:374–384
3. Katayama H et al (1990) Adverse reaction to ionic and non-ionic CM. Radiology 175:621–628

Table 4.15.1. Prevalence of ADRs by age Distribution (from [3])

Age of patient (years)	Cases with ionic contrast media			Cases with nonionic contrast media		
	Total (n)	With ADR (n) (%)	With severe ADR (n) (%)	Total (n)	With ADR (n) (%)	With severe ADR (n) (%)
< 1	272	2 (0.74)	0 (0)	916	4 (0.44)	0 (0)
1– 9	2 701	338 (12.51)	2 (0.07)	5 479	138 (2.52)	4(0.07)
10–19	6 359	1 068 (16.80)	26 (0.41)	7 066	319 (4.51)	5 (0.07)
20–29	8 842	1 615 (18.27)	21 (0.24)	8 009	372 (4.64)	5 (0.06)
30–39	16 428	2 806 (17.08)	49 (0.30)	14 569	661 (4.54)	6 (0.04)
40–49	25 352	3 825 (15.09)	69 (0.27)	23 386	962 (4.11)	13 (0.06)
50–59	40 311	5 025 (12.47)	69 (0.17)	38 014	1 200 (3.16)	15 (0.04)
60–69	38 807	4 087 (10.53)	82 (0.21)	38 220	996 (2.61)	10 (0.03)
70–79	24 807	2 185 (8.81)	41 (0.17)	26 201	507 (1.94)	8 (0.03)
≥ 80	4 681	371 (7.93)	6 (0.13)	5 562	81 (1.46)	4 (0.07)
No entry	724	...	...	941	...	...

4. Katayama H et al (1991) Full-scale investigation into adverse reaction in Japan, risk factor analysis. Invest Radiol 26 [Suppl]:S1–S4
5. Shehadi WH (1975) Adverse reactions to intravasculary administered CM. AJR 124:115–152
6. Shehadi WH et al (1980) Adverse reactions to CM. Radiology 137:299–302
7. Shehadi WH (1985) Acta Radiol Diagn 26:457–461

4.16 Does Weather Influence the Rate of Undesirable Reactions to Contrast Media Administration?

D. Zuckert

The effects of certain weather conditions on the human autonomic nervous system are known: cold-air advective states primarily activate the sympathetic nervous system, whereas warm-air advective states activate the vagus.

Even though enough evidence has been gathered showing the effects of meteorological conditions on the human organism in the form of increased occurrence of such pathological conditions as thromboembolism and dysregulation, for the time being the discussion of mechanisms of their pathogenesis must remain speculative.

In a comprehensive study from 1979 to 1981, it proved possible to establish connections between the frequency of the occurrence of CM side effects and definite meteorological conditions present at the time. Thus, there is some justification for assuming that both weather coming from the east and low-pressure fronts with rising air movements favour the occurrence of CM incidents. Under these conditions, we found a side-effect frequency rate of up to 11% following conventional CM. Under the influence of a high-pressure system and in markedly cold-air advective meteorological states, on the other hand, incidents were less frequent, namely 4.7% and 5.3%, respectively.

The pathogenesis of CM incidents nevertheless remains largely unclear for the moment, even though very intensive research has been made into many individual factors such as histamine release, complement activation, the coagulation system, functional disorders of the central nervous system and psychological influences. All these factors may play a part, though their definitive roles have not yet been clarified in detail. Nor can the relationship of meteorological phenomena to the frequency of CM side effects be attributed to any single factor, since the effects of individual meteorological parameters on humans has not yet been sufficiently clarified. However, studies show that the particular reactive state of the individual patient at the time of the examination certainly plays an important role, not only in terms of the meteorological situation as a whole, but also in reference to subjective sensitivity to weather conditions.

4.17 Can Contrast Media Procedures Be Carried Out Despite Defined Risks?

P. Dawson

In the author's opinion there are no absolute contraindications to contrast-enhanced studies. Risk and contraindication in medicine, as elsewhere, are always relative terms. Clearly, if there is a definable factor increasing the risk of the procedure, thought must be given to whether it is really necessary and to whether an alternative and possible safer procedure not requiring CM might give the same or similar information. In the patient in whom, in spite of definable risk factors, a contrast examination is still thought necessary, several precautions may be taken: nonionic CM should be used since these are associated with a reduced incidence of reactions, particularly in high risk patients [1] and are associated with reduced toxicity in higher doses [2]; the smallest dose compatible with obtaining the essential information should be used; prophylaxis with corticosteroids or antihistamines should be given to patients who have reacted on a previous occasion, are atopic or asthmatic, or are generally allergic to other drugs or agents. An anaesthesist might be asked to present in case of the need for skilled resuscitation.

Only the clinician in charge of the case with full knowledge of the individual patient's clinical history and current state of health can properly assess the situation and no precise rules of conduct can reasonably be laid down. If the radiologist has sensibly considered the need for the examination, excluded the possibility that alternative methods might provide the information needed, has assessed the likely risk as far as is possible and has taken some of the precautions listed above, then he will have acted reasonably both ethically and medico-legally speaking.

References

1. Dawson P, Hemingway A (1987) Contrast doses in interventional radiology. J Intervent Radiol 2:145–146
2. Katayama H et al (1990) Report of the Japanese committee on the safety of contrast media. Radiology 175:621–628

4.18 What Interactions Are Known Between the Administration of Contrast Media and Other Medications?

P. Dawson

A number of drugs are known to be physically incompatible with some CM [3]. These incompatibilities include persistent or transient precipitation with conventional and low osmolality CM of papaverine, protamine, cimetidine, diphenhydramin-HCl and garamycin. No such incompatibilities are known with the nonionic agents but great caution should be exercised in the physical mixing of any drugs prior to injection into patients.

A number of drugs have been tested in animals in clinical range doses to investigate the possibility of synergism with radiocontrast agents. Among the commonly used drugs, only the cardiac glycosides have been found to act synergistically [1]. Another observation was that Strophanthin-K in the near lethal dose range produced a greater mortality if low or clinical doses if Diatrizoate were given with it [1]. Fischer and colleagues [1] also noted synergism between nonionic metrizamide and cardiac glycosides with cardiopulmonary death. Since many of the toxic effects of the glycosides are on the heart with arrythmias and ventricular fibrillation in high doses, it is not surprising that CM, which have their own cardiotoxic effects may act synergistically with these. However, there is some evidence that the effects are centrally mediated rather than directly on the heart [5].

Hamilton has reported two patients taking β-blockers who suffered hypotensive reactions while undergoing excretory urography [2]. Perhaps the β-adrenergic blocking agents may interfere with the body's ability to counteract hypotension-inducing events such as those associated with CM. It might also be thought, though there is no clinical evidence, that there may be a possibility of a synergistic effect as regards bronchospasm in susceptible patients between β-blockers and CM.

A synergistic effect between the calcium antagonist verapamil and ionic CM has been observed in experimental coronary angiography as an enhanced inhibition of atrioventricular conduction [4]. No such effects have been observed following peripheral injection of CM experimentally or clinically.

The possibility that angiotensin-converting enzyme (ACE) inhibitors might act synergistically with CM has been raised [5]. Both inhibit ACE and could, theoretically, lead to high levels of bradykinin in association with contrast administration. This remains entirely speculative.

One well-established synergy is between the first generation nonionic agent metrizamide administered intrathecally and concomitant systemic chlorpromazine [5]. No significant interactions have been established involving the second generation nonionic agents.

References

1. Fischer MW, Morris TW, King AN, Harnish PP (1978) Deleterious synergism of a cardiac glycoside and sodium diatrizoate. Investigative Radiology 1978, 13:340–346
2. Hamilton G. Severe adverse reactions to urography in patients taking β-adrenergic blocking agents. Canadian Medical Association Journal 1985, 133:122
3. Irving MD, Burbridge BE (1989) Incompatibility of contrast agents with intravascular medications. Radiology 173:91–92
4. Lasser EC (1987) A general and personal perspective on contrast material research. Invest Radiol 23:S71–S74
5. Maly P, Olivecrona M, Almen T, Golman K (1984) Interaction between chlorpromazine and intrathecally injected non-ionics contrast media in non-anaesthetised rabbits. Neuroradiology 26:235–240
6. Peck WW, Slutsky RA, Mancini J, Higgins CB. Combined actions of verapamil and contrast media on atrio-ventricular conduction. Invest Radiol 19:202–207

4.19 What Is the Role of X-Ray Contrast Media Administered During Pregnancy or in Nursing Mothers?

H. Imhof and
K. Vergesslich

Since the introduction of nonionic CM the occurrence of adverse side effects has been markedly reduced. Therefore these CM are widely used in paediatric radiology practice, even in newborn infants. However, the question about CM administration during pregnancy and in nursing mothers is still controversial.

Because of the small amounts entering the fetal or infant circulation, side effects involving kidney or liver function do not have to be taken into consideration. In addition, low osmolality of the current CM prevents severe disturbance of the osmolality equilibrium in the fragile fetus or newborn infant.

The thyroid function of the fetus, however, may be significantly altered by iodine containing CM passing freely through the placental barrier. The same phenomenon can be observed in newborn infants. It is well known that iodine blood levels increase exponentially after intravenous administration of CM in this age group. The iodine excess can cause hypothyroidism. Though this is usually a transient phenomenon, the effect on the maturing infant brain is unclear and possible deleterious effects cannot unequivocally be ruled out. After administration of iodine-containing X-ray CM for amniofoetography, hypothyroidism has been observed in several newborn infants [1].

Thus, the following statements can be made:

1. The administration of CM during pregnancy should only be performed for essential indications. Close monitoring of thyroid function after birth is mandatory in the newborn.

2. When nursing, the milk should not be fed until three days after the examination.

References

1. Stubbe P, Heidemann P, Schürnbrand P et al (1980) Eur J Ped 135:97

CHAPTER 5

Prophylactic Measures

5.1	**What Is the Place of Fasting and Dehydration Before Contrast Media Administration?**

W. Clauß

Since risk patients tolerate nonionic X-ray CM and effective premedications are available, previously frequent side effects of CM examinations, such as nausea and vomiting, now occur rarely. Moreover, patients who have not had anything to eat or drink for longer periods of time are less calm and cooperative and more susceptible to side effects during an examination. In view of this, in 1992 a German group of radiological experts took up the question of optimal patient preparation, in the interests of both physician and patient and for the safety of the latter. A survey of the participating experts showed great discrepancies in the recommended periods of abstinence from solid food and liquids prior to intraarterial, intravenous, intrathecal, and intraarticular CM administration (Fig. 5.1.1 a–d); standardization therefore seemed desirable. After intensive, as well as con-

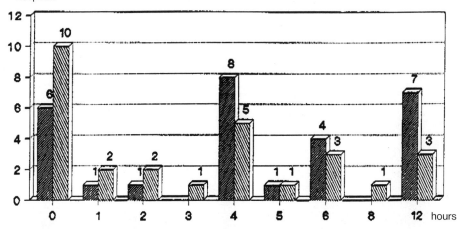

hospitals

Fig. 5.1.1a–d. Intra-arterial (**a**), intravenous (**b**), intrathecal (**c**), and intra-articular (**d**) CM administration: abstinence from solid food and liquids. ■, abstinence from solid food; ▨, abstinence from liquids

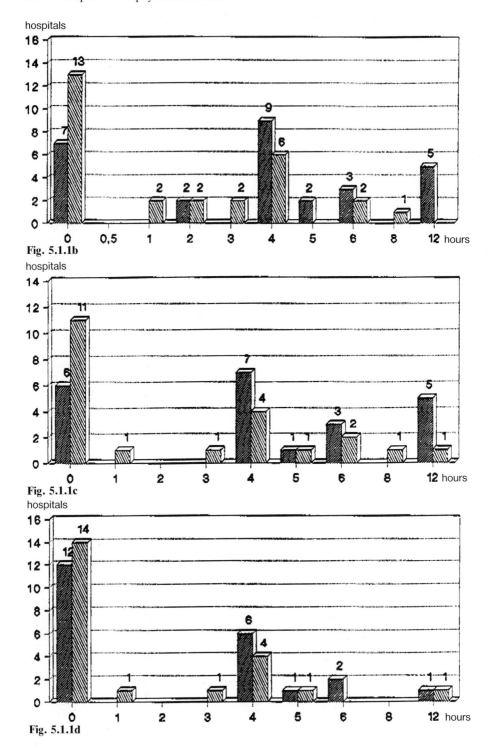

Fig. 5.1.1b

Fig. 5.1.1c

Fig. 5.1.1d

troversial discussions, a recommendation was made to hydrate patients adequately both before and after CM administration, i.e. to urge the patient to drink. Moreover, for the administration of nonionic X-ray CM, sufficient reasons could no longer be found for maintaining the previously held recommendation of at least a 4-h absolute abstinence from food.

A small meal taken before most examinations (the size of which, however, should be agreed upon in consultation with the anaesthetist) often decreases the strain of the examination for both physician and patient [1].

References

1. Expertengespräch Kontrastmittel (1992) Radiologe 9 (Suppl)

5.2 Can Hypersensitivity Reactions to Contrast Media Be Predicted Through Preliminary Testing?

W. Clauß and *V. Taenzer*

It used to be common in clinical practice to carry out subcutaneous, intradermal, conjunctival or intravascular testing with small doses of CM, in order to detect possible hypersensitivity. It turned out, however, that the skin test and even the intravenous testing yielded very unreliable results. Whereas positive results of such hypersensitivity tests were often followed by completely symptomless tolerance of the subsequently administered CM, severe and even lethal reactions could sometimes be observed in examinations subsequent to negative test results. The uncertainty in interpreting preliminary testing results, combined with the experience that even the small amounts of CM administered intravascularly in such testing, could trigger severe anaphylactoid reactions resulting in death, led to the 1967 resolution of the Congress of European Radiologists to stop preliminary testing in CM administration. Since this time, refraining from CM testing neither represents malpractive nor does it possess any medico-legal implications.

Today one assumes that antigen-antibody reactions, which can be detected in preliminary testing, are not involved in reactions of hypersensitivity to CM. Therefore, prophylactic measures aimed at reducing such hypersensitivity reactions, the possibility of which can never be excluded, and rapid therapeutic intervention for treating them remain important in any administration of CM.

5.3 Is Sedation Indicated Before Administering Contrast Media?

G. Wisser

Anxiety is frequently viewed as inducing undesirable reactions to

CM administration. In a survey in 1983, 82% of almost 1500 radiologists believed that fear is the most frequent cause of mild, undesirable reactions; 37% even considered it the main cause of more severe reactions, such as shock, pulmonary and cardiovascular problems and deaths [5].

In 1980, Lalli put forward the hypothesis that all CM reactions are triggered by a direct effect of the CM on the CNS. Fear and anxiety are seen here as functioning as emotional triggers [4]. He was able to show that the occurrence of nausea, vomiting and urticaria was significantly reduced through hypnotic influence prior to CM administration. In contrast, diazepam significantly increased the incidence of such mild reactions [3]. Patients who became more anxious as a result of discussions prior to CM administration did not, however, show a statistically significant increase in undesirable reactions [6].

Today, immunological (allergic, anaphylactic) and nonimmunological (pseudoallergic, anaphylactoid) reactions are considered the pathomechanisms of CM incidents [7] and one has to advise against the exclusive administration of sedatives as prophylaxis. In patients at risk (patients with known allergies; cardiac, pulmonary or hepatic disease; bronchial asthma; exposure to CM within the last few days), nonionic CM possibly supplemented by corticoids and/or antihistamines should be used. Sedation prior to CM administration may, however, be considered in states of agitation [2] or in order to avoid vasovagal reactions [1].

References

1. Bielory L, Kaliner MA (1985) Anaphylactoid reactions to radiocontrast materials. Int Anesthesiol Clin 23:97–118
2. Elke M, Brune K (1980) Prophylaktische Maßnahmen vor Kontrastmittelinjektionen. Dtsch med Wschr 105:250–252
3. Lalli AF (1974) Urographic contrast media reactions and anxiety. Radiology 112:267–271
4. Lalli AF (1980) Contrast media reactions: data analysis and hypothesis. Radiology 134:1–12
5. Spring DB, Akin JR, Margulis AR (1984) Informed consent for intravenous contrast-enhanced radiography: a national survey of practice and opinion. Radiology 152:609–613
6. Spring DB, Winfield AC, Friedland GW, Shuman WP, Preger L (1989) Written informed consent for iv contrast-enhanced radiography – Reply. Amer J Roentgenol 153:189
7. Wangemann BU, Jantzen JP, Dick W (1988) Anästhesiologische Aspekte allergischer Reaktionen am Beispiel des „Kontrastmittelzwischenfalls". Anaesth Intensivmed 29:205–214

5.4 Does General Anaesthesia Prevent the Occurrence of Contrast Media-Induced Side Effects?

G. Wisser

General anaesthesia has been frequently recommended for angiographic examinations, especially those involving ionic CM. It was claimed that it not only facilitates the diagnostic procedure (e.g. elimination of CM-induced pain and defence mechanisms and restlessness on part of the patient), but that it also had a protective effect against undesirable CM reactions [4, 6].

Prospective, randomized, comparative studies on undesirable side effects do not exist. Due to the nature of general anaesthesia, mild reactions to CM, such as nausea, vomiting, etc., cannot even be observed [8]. CM-induced skin reactions occur equally often whether the patient is conscious or under anaesthesia [1]; there is not even a demonstrable difference in frequency in CM-induced hypotension in general or spinal anaesthesia [8]. Even the most severe reactions (anaphylactic-anaphylactoid shock) have been observed under anaesthesia for both ionic [2, 5, 7] and nonionic CM [3, 10].

Thus, general anaesthesia does not provide absolute protection against a CM incident. Accordingly, the question of whether anaesthesia is indicated should be decided in terms of an assessment of the individual risks. Mere knowledge of a CM risk factor does not justify anaesthesia [9]. According to our present state of knowledge, general anaesthesia cannot be recommended as an alternative to prophylaxis with corticoids and/or antihistaminic preparations in the prevention of potential CM incidents.

References

1. Albrecht K (1956) Das Risiko bei neurochirurgischen Untersuchungsmethoden. Zentralbl Chir 81:2107–2113
2. Gottlieb A, Lalli AF (1982) Hypotension following contrast media injection during general anesthesia. Anesth Analg 61:387–389
3. Jantzen JPA, Wangemann B, Wisser G (1989) Adverse reactions to non-ionic iodinated contrast media do occu

during general anesthesia. Anesthesiology 70:561
4. Maus H, Loennecken SJ (1962) Zerebrale Angiographie und Narkose. Fortschr Neurol Psychiatr 30:155–165
5. Pfeifer G, Solymosi L, Grimm R, Wappenschmidt J (1984) Anästhesie in der Neuroradiologie. Anaesth Intensivther Notfallmed 19:57–59
6. Plötz J, Viehweger G (1974) Die Angiographie der oberen Extremität in Narkose, lokaler und regionaler Anästhesie. Prakt Anaest 9:225–231
7. Simmendinger HJ, Just OH (1973) Anaphylaktischer Schock nach Kontrastmittelinjektion. Z prakt Anaest 8:370–374
8. Tolksdorf W, Raddi U, Rohowsky R, Lutz H (1980) Zur Wahl des Anästhesieverfahrens bei translumbalen Aortographien. Anaesth Intensivther Notfallmed 15:400–406
9. Wangemann BU, Wisser G (1990) Prophylaxe des „Kontrastmittelzwischenfalls" durch Allgemeinanästhesie? Radiologe 30:141–144
10. Wisser G, Wangemann B, Jantzen JP, Dick W (1990) Anaphylaktoide Reaktion auf ein nichtionisches Röntgenkontrastmittel in Allgemeinanästhesie. Anaesth Intensiv Ther Notfallmed 25:271–273

5.5 Can the Rate of Contrast Media-Induced Side Effects Be Lowered by Premedication with Antihistamines?

R. Tauber

A substantial proportion of CM side effects are probably induced by histamine. Thus, on the one hand, a rise in the plasma histamine level can be observed after CM administration, and on the other, histamine-induced side effects can be prevented by a prophylaxis with H_1- and H_2-receptor antagonists.

However, it must always be taken into account that histamine H_1- and H_2-receptor blockers only block histamine-induced side effects and therefore only cover part of the possible spectrum of pathogenesis. Other reaction pathways in the complement, coagulation and immune systems are not blocked.

Nevertheless, if risk factors exist that increase the danger of X-ray CM side effects, these patients should receive, premedication with H_1- and H_2-receptor antagonist. These are patients:

– With an allergic diathesis, with hypersensitivity to food and drugs, and those undergoing blood transfusions
– Who have already reacted to CM in the past
– With diseases accompanied by raised histamine levels, e.g. pulmonary diseases
– Who are elderly (over 75 years old) or are children
– With cardiac, respiratory, or hepatic insufficiency.

The intravenous injection of H_1- and H_2-receptor antagonists has to be 10–15 min before CM administration; injection should be over for 2 min.

As an H_1 antagonist, dimethindene maleate can be used (Fenistil; 4 mg for a body wt. of 40–60 kg, 8 mg for a body wt. of 60–100 kg, and 12 mg for a body wt. over 100 kg). As an H_2 antagonist, cimetidine can be used (Tagamet; 200 mg for a body wt. of 40–60 kg, 400 mg for a body wt. of 60–100 kg, and 600 mg for a body wt. over 100 kg).

If patients are correctly premedicated, one can perform urography without the presence of an anaesthetist. Even in cases of known CM intolerance, excretory urography need not be performed under anaesthesia. Full resuscitation facilities must, however, always be available.

5.6 Can the Adverse Reaction Rate/Be Reduced by Administration of Corticosteroids?

W. Clauß

In patients with known CM hypersensitivity and in those who suffer from allergy, a two- to six-fold rise in the side-effect rate has to be reckoned with following intravascular CM administration. Reactions are largely independent of doses and are categorized as pseudoanaphylaxis.

The administration of corticosteroids has been recommended since the 1960s as a prophylactic measure. Neither the pathomechanisms of anaphylactoid involved in the genesis of pseudoanaphylaxis nor the mechanisms operating in corticosteroid prevention or reduction of these reactions have been fully elaborated. However, in vitro tests have displayed some features of corticosteroids that could be drawn upon in clarifying its effects. Thus, they counteract experimentally produced permeability impairment of cell membranes [7], check the complement-induced lysis of erythrocytes [4], lower the serum-complement level [1] and counteract both the release of histamine from mast cells [3] and haemolysis [6].

The unsatisfactory prophylactic effect of corticoisteroids given intravenously immediately prior to CM administration has been explained in terms of the slow onset of their effects. Results can be improved by increasing the interval (several hours) between the administration of corticosteroid and that of the CM. Recourse can also be made to quick-acting corticosteroids, such as triamcinolone acetonide phosphate disodium salt (Volon A solubile) [2]. In recent years, the good prophylactic effects of oral corticosteroids that are fractionated and administered over a longer period of time has been attested to. For example, the two-part, oral administration of 32 mg each of methylprednisolone 12 h and 2 h prior to CM administration leads to a significant lowering of the side-effect rate [5]. Even though prophylaxis this regime of preceding the administration of ionic CM leads to a lower rate of side effects, this rate is still higher than the side-effect rate resulting from the administration of nonionic CM without preceding corticoid administration [8].

References

1. Atkinson JP et al (1973) Effect of cortisone therapy on serum complement components. J Immunol 111:1061–1066
2. Fiegel G (1985) Vermeiden von Kontrastmittelzwischenfällen. Med Welt 36:1486–1470
3. Greaves MW et al (1974) Glucocorticoid inhibition of antigen-evoked histamine release from human skin. Immunolgy 27:359–364
4. Jennings JF et al (1966) The effect of hydrocortisone on immune lysis of cells induced by cytotoxic antibody and complement in vitro. J Immunol 96:409–414
5. Lasser EC et al (1977) Theoretical and experimental basis for utilization in prevention of contrast media reactions. Radiology 125:1–9
6. Schreiber AD et al (1975) Effect of corticosteroids on the human monocyte IgG and complement receptors. J Clin Invest 56:1189–1197
7. Weissman G (1961) Release of lysosomal protease by ultraviolet irradiation and inhibition by hydrocortisone. Exp Cell Res 25:207–210
8. Wolf GL (1989) Adverse reactions to intravenous contrast media in routine clinical practice. Scientific Poster, RSNA 1989

CHAPTER 6

Informing the Patient Prior to Contrast Media Administration

6.1 What Is the Patients "Right to Know" Prior to an X-Ray Examination Using Contrast Media?

H. J. Maurer
and *W. Spann*

(The following section was prepared in the context of German law. Many of the basic principles are of universal application though, naturally, caution should be exercised.)

Even though no detailed legal regulations exist, informing the patient about the nature and possible risks of a diagnostic examination has always been an indispensable part of all preparation. If such examinations or interventions are performed on a patient who is not adequately informed, they are not in accordance with the law. Only if
a) the examination is indicated,
b) the intervention is performed according to the state of the art, and
c) the patient's consent to the intervention is legally valid
is the examination in accordance with the law.

Consent is considered legally valid only if it was given with clear understanding of the situation, i.e. if it was informed consent. The patient can only gain such clear understanding of the situation of his or her specific case by being informed by a physician. Accordingly, adequately informing the patient is a necessary condition of the lawfulness of consent and thus of the procedure as well.

During such a consultation the experienced physician can take the opportunity to reassure the patient, reduce his fear of the examination and win his trust. Anxious patients do not merely make the diagnostic procedure more difficult through lack of cooperation; when they are administered CM, the physician must reckon with a higher rate of side effects [1].

If legal proceedings are initiated due to the failure to inform adequately, the burden of proof rests upon the physician. For this reason, it is necessary at all times to be able to prove that the patient was informed, be it in the form of his or her signature, witnesses, and/or an entry into the medical file. In the same way, written record must be kept if the patient waives his or her right to be informed or if he or she has no further questions regarding the examination or its attendant risks.

In legal terms, the placing of a catheter and the injection of a CM qualify as bodily injury. For this reason, every recognized danger or recognized risk connected to the given diagnostic intervention has to be explained to the patient, regardless of the frequency of its occurrence. At least under German law, the referring physician is also partly responsible for informing the patient [2].

Patients must not just be informed prior to the procedure; they must be given an adequate opportunity to think it over. In invasive, diagnostic procedures (e.g. angiography), the discussion should be conducted on the day preceding the examination. Patients may be informed on the day of the examination in the case of urography or CT; however, this should occur some time prior to the procedure and outside the examination room.

The patient should be informed far enough in advance of any examination reduction in driving fitness, so that he or she does not drive to the examination.

In the case of unconscious or unresponsive patients (emergencies), the physician has to perform the necessary examination without informing the patient. He or she can work on the basis of presumed consent and represents in such cases the interests of the patient in addition to his or her own.

Consent for the examination must be obtained from both parents when the patient (for example, a child) does not fully understand the situation. If this is not possible, then the person who has custody of the child must give permission. If the parents refuse to give consent in a life-threatening situation and there is no time to obtain consent of court, the physician should conduct the examination anyway.

When explaining to a patient the risks involved in a diagnostic examination the physician should draw primarily on his own experience. It might also be helpful to be able to provide statistics from other examiners. The patient also has a right to know about the various rates of CM side effects (for example, ionic and nonionic CM). Price alone should not influence a physician's decision.

Outpatients should be informed of rare but possible late reactions as well as of any effects CM might have on driving a motor vehicle.

References

1. Lalli AF (1974) Urographic contrast media reactions and anxiety. Radiology 112:267–271
2. Maurer HJ, Clauß W, Granitza A (1983) Alleinige oder geteilte Verantwortlichkeit bei der Anwendung jodierter Röntgenkontrastmittel. Röntgen-BL 36:379–383

6.2 What Special Information Should a Healthy Volunteer/Patient Receive Who Is Participating in a Clinical Study of a New Drug?

W. Clauß and *E. Andrew*

Volunteers patients participating in clinical studies have not only rights but also duties that should be conveyed to them in a comprehensive and understandable fashion both verbally and in writing (volunteer/patient information).

The planning and execution of a clinical study, including obtaining the informed consent of the volunteer/patient is subject to the laws of the land and to the European "Good Clinical Practice" (GCP) Guidelines (11.07. 1990 version). Moreover, the recommendations of the World Medical Association should be taken into account (revised declaration of Helsinki in the Hong Kong version, 1988).

Aside from being informed in writing, the volunteer/patient also has the right to question the physician on all points of the clinical study. The volunteer/patient declares his voluntary participation in the knowledge that he can withdraw his consent at any time without having to suffer any disadvantage in the course of subsequent treatment.

Volunteer/patient information has, above all, to take the following points into account:

- Participation in the study has to be justified and alternative methods of treatment indicated to the volunteer/patient.
- Participation is voluntary and can be discontinued at any time without explanation.
- The study involves the testing of a drug not yet admitted to the market.
- A description must be given of the effects already known or suspected, tolerability and side-effect rates (frequency and degree of severity) of the drug. If no clinical experience exists with the drug whatsoever, then preclinical results have to be consulted.
- A description must be given of the state of development of the preparation and of the general goal of the individual study.
- The test design (open, single- or double-blind) must be explained and a description of the course of the study (preparatory phase, test-induced study length, follow-up phase) ist to be provided.
- A description of additional demands of the study (diet, blood samples, prohibited accompanying medications, confinement to bed and so forth) must be provided.
- Information must be provided about taking out an insurance policy covering possible examination-induced morbidity. The threat to insurance coverage that is entailed by not immediately reporting side effects or by consenting to additional, simultaneous treatments without the knowledge of the study physician must be pointed out.
- The confidential treatment of the resulting test data and the strict protection of personal data, even in the case of monitoring by supervisory agencies, must be pointed out.

Clinical studies on children and on mentally disturbed patients is only permissible if the tested preparation is being developed specially for the diagnosis and/or therapy of certain diseases of these groups or if results obtained from other groups of patients are not applicable to these groups.

CHAPTER 7

Administration of Contrast Media

7.1 Are Contrast Media Heated to Body Temperature Better Tolerated?

P. Dawson

It seems, from first principles, entirely reasonable that CM which are, generally speaking, injected into patients in high concentrations and large doses might be better tolerated if delivered at body temperature. Many radiologists use one of the commercially available thermostatically controlled heating cabinets to warm their CM to 37°C. In any case, toxicity and tolerance aside, warming the CM to body temperature significantly reduces its viscosity, making injection easier, particularly with small needles and catheters [1].

There is, however, little hard evidence available to support the idea that clinical tolerance is significantly increased thereby. The only recent reasonably large study (but still only 100 patients) revealed no convincing difference between two patient groups, one receiving room temperature CM and the other receiving body temperature CM [2].

It is interesting to note that as regards pain and heat sensation specifically in arteriography, there does appear to be an association with CM viscosity and at least some evidence, therefore, that these undesirable side effects may be diminished by heating the CM [3]. The evidence, however, comes from comparative studies of different CM with different viscosities and not from studies with the same CM at different viscosities (different temperatures) so other factors than viscosity might well be confusing the picture.

In summary, supporting evidence of benefit is lacking, but heating CM to body temperature before use is being more and more widely practised and, in the author's opinion, is to be recommended.

References

1. Halsell RD (1987) Heating contrast media in role contemporary angiography. Radiology 164:276–278
2. Turner E, Kentner P, Melamed JL, Rao G, Seitz MJ (1982) Frequency of anaphylactoid reactions during intravenous urography with radiographic contrast media at two different temperatures. Radiology 143:327–329
3. Wilcox J, Sage MR (1984) Is viscosity important in the production of blood-brain-barrier disruption by intracarotid contrast media? Neuroradiology 26:511–513?

7.2 Are There Any Guidelines for Maximum Doses in Angiography?

P. Dawson

Iodinated CM are mild tissue poisons generally used in large doses. Because even the low osmolality agents represent a potential osmotic load stress to a patient, attention must be paid to the total dose given and to the time course over which it is given. Guidelines, sometimes given in terms of ml per kilogram of patient, are vague since the strength of the solution is not stated. Milligrams iodine per kilogram (mg I/kg) is the clearest notation since the radiologist usually has some feel for iodine doses and concentrations but he must still do some calculations to find what volume of solution he may use. Some examples will now be given but should not be taken as prescriptive:

1. An IVU is frequently performed with approx 300 mg I/kg. In a 70 kg man this is 21 000 mg I (21 g). If a solution of 420 mg I/ml is used ([e.g. "Conray 420"] the volume required is 21 000/420 = 50 ml (one bottle)
2. A "high dose" IVU might utilize 600 mg I/kg, i.e. two bottles of 420 mg I/ml strength
3. An angiogram might easily require 1000 mg I/kg of patient. If, say, a solution of 350 mg I/ml were utilized thus would be equivalent, in a 70 kg man, to: 1000 × 70/350 = 200 ml (= four bottles).

Such a dose might be considered by many as much as is prudent to give to most patients, but there is no doubt that more is given on occasion in complex angiography. Naturally, there are some patients at greater absolute or relative risk – small infants, frail elderly patients, patients with cardiac or renal disease, for example – and doses have to be reduced in recognition of these. Working on the basis of known toxicities we can reasonably suppose that whatever is taken as the upper limit "allowed" in any given patient may be doubled, in terms of iodine dose, if a nonionic rather than a conventional ionic agent is used. Digital systems are helpful when available because they allow images to be obtained with dilute CM, thereby reducing total dose.

7.3 Are There Any Guidelines for Maximum Doses in Myelography?

I. O. Skalpe

Following the introduction of the nonionic CM iohexol (Omnipaque) for myelography, complications which can be ascribed to the CM occur very rarely. Nevertheless, one should keep the dose as low as possible for establishing the diagnosis. We have never found it necessary to exceed a maximum dose of 3 g I (10 ml CM at 300 mg I/ml) and recommend this as a maximum dose in adults.

Children have a high tolerance for iohexol in myelography. One should bear in mind that the spinal sub-arachnoid space is, relatively speaking, larger in children than in adults. Therefore, in relation to body weight, higher doses are necessary in children than in adults. We suggest the following guidelines for maximum doses in children: below 1 year of age 5 ml CM at 180 mg I/ml; 1–4 years 5 ml CM at 240 mg I/ml; 4–12 years 8 ml CM at 240 mg I/ml. Above the age of 12 the same doses as in adults may be used.

7.4 Are There Any Guidelines for Maximum Doses in Cholegraphy?

V. Taenzer

Biliary elimination of CM is limited by the functional capacity of hepatocytes. In humans, the biliary transport maximum for the biliary CM, meglumine iotroxate (Biliscopin), lies around 0.35 mg I min/kg. This implies that in cholegraphy, as opposed to urography, there is only a very limited dose range up to the transport maximum and up to which dose increases will have the desired effect of raising CM concentration in the bile. Further dose increases only lead to heterotopic CM excretion via the kidneys. Adjusted to the biliary transport maximum, a dose of 20–30 ml cholegraphic CM in a concentration of 180 mg/ml (Biliscopin) has proved to be the maximum effective CM dose.

7.5 Can "Maximum" Doses Be Exceeded?

P. Dawson

In considering dose-related CM toxicity it is important to realize that there are two different aspects. Firstly, there is evidence that ana-phylactoid reactions are, to some extent, dose related [1]. It is true that they may occur following injection of a very small dose, even subcutaneously, but, for the most part, appear to be associated with injections of significant volumes intravascularly [1]. Secondly, there is the question of high dose toxicity [2]. As regards this, the problem is to define "high dose" and, more difficult yet, to define "maximum permissible" dose. Everything will clearly be patient dependent and will be dependent on the time period during which the total dose is to be given. Clearly, what would be quite moderate doses for some patients might be disastrous for those with impaired cardiac reserve and, equally clearly, while several hundred millilitres of a CM might be acceptable if given in a complex interventional procedure over a period of 2 or 3 h, it would not be acceptable if given by rapid intravenous injection over a period of less than 1 min.

Some general guidelines may be given:

Those at risk from what might be described as contrast overdose in absolute terms include small infants undergoing complex angiocardiographic procedures and otherwise healthy patients undergoing prolonged and complex interventional procedures [2]. Those at risk from what might be described as relative CM overdose include patients with poor cardiac reserve and with poor renal function [2]. Low osmolality agents in general, and nonionic agents in particular, are to be preferred in any cases where absolute or relative CM overdose may be anticipated [2]. The use of these agents does not, however, guarantee total safety, but animal toxicity studies do appear to demonstrate that nonionic agents ought to offer a margin of safety in terms of total dose of some three times.

No dogmatic statements can be made in this area but, if the procedure is necessary and if the CM is used carefully in order to minimize the total dose, then, in the context of the particular patient concerned, his general physical condition and the urgency of diagnosis and/or interventional treatment of the disease, then some three times what ever maximum iodine dose is considered permissible with a conventional agent may be used in the form of a nonionic CM.

However, renal function is always a concern when high doses of CM are used and the status of the nonionic agents in this regard has not been clearly established. Caution is therefore necessary and monitoring of renal function after a high dose procedure recommended.

References

1. Ansell G (1987) Radiological contrast media. In: Inman WHW (ed) Monitoring for drug safety, 2nd ed. MTP Press, Lancashire, pp 337–348

2. Dawson P, Hemingway A (1987) Contrast doses in interventional radiology. J Intervent Radiol 2:145–146

7.6 Does the Injection Rate Affect the Tolerance?

P. Dawson

If a drug is to be injected in large volumes and doses, as is often the case with intravascular CM, then one naturally assumes that rapid injections would be less well tolerated than slower injections. The report by Shehadi in 1975 [5] that in his large series of intravascular CM administrations there was a lower incidence of adverse effects in injections taking less than 2 min than in those taking from 3–10 min was somewhat surprising. He found, incidentally, the reverse to be the case for intravenous cholangiography.

Davies et al. [2] observed, on the other hand, an increase in sensation of warmth with rapid injections but otherwise no difference in the rate of side effects in comparison with slower injection over 2 min or so.

Animal experiments involving the rapid injection of large doses of CM have indicated a considerable increase in toxicity [1]. Whereas the $LD_{50\%}$ of sodium diatrizoate by slow intravenous injection in the dog was 13.2 g/kg of animal, with rapid injection the $LD_{50\%}$ dropped to 2.7 g/kg of animal.

Pfister and Hutter [4] furthermore observed that the incidence of electrocardiographic changes during intravenous urography was related to the rapidity of injection.

Lorenz has pointed out that drugs which cause histamine release (this includes CM) are more likely to do so if given by more rapid bolus injection than by slow infusion [3].

Therefore, notwithstanding Shehadi's interesting observation [5] made in the context of an excellent and well-regarded large-scale study, the weight of clinical and experimental evidence appears to suggest that rapid injections are less desirable than slower injections. Certainly, it would appear reasonable to suggest that in the more susceptible older patients, or in those with known cardiac disease, a slower injection would be safe where this is consistent with diagnostic demands.

References

1. Bernstein EF, Palmer JD, Aaberg TA, Davis RL (1961) Studies on the toxicology of Hypaque-90% following rapid venous injection. Radiology 76:88–95
2. Davies P, Roberts MB, Roylance J (1975) Acute reactions to urographic contrast media. BMJ 2:434–437
3. Lorenz W, Doericke A (1985) Histamino libération induite par les produits anésthesique ou leurs solvants: spécifique ou non-spécifique. Ann Fr Anesth Reanim 4:115–123
4. Pfister RC, Hutter AM (1982) Alteration in heart rate and rhythm at urography with sodium diatrizoate. Acta Radiologica 23:107–110
5. Shehadi WM (1975) Adverse reactions to intravascularly administered contrast media. AJR 124:145–152

7.7 What Fluids Can be Recommended for Flushing Catheters?

P. Dawson

Blood coming into contact with foreign surfaces such as catheters is activated to clot with a consequent risk of thromboembolism if such a clot is reinjected into the patient. Catheters must therefore be flushed frequently, and this is perhaps the most important aspect of angiographic technique [3]. Any physiologically acceptable solution may be used to achieve this object – sterile water, saline, heparinized saline, or CM, for example. In the past CM themselves, because of their known anticoagulant effects, were sometimes recommended as flushing solutions [4]. This area has become confused recently, and the confidence of angiographers somewhat eroded, by controversy surrounding the haematological properties of nonionic CM [2, 6]. Suggestions have been made that these agents are in some way procoagulant. There is in fact no basis for this assertion and all the evidence points to the fact that they are, like their ionic counterparts, entirely anticoagulant in effect [1]. They are simply less anticoagulant than the ionic agents and therefore not as effective in this role. This point having been made, however, there is no positive reason why they should not be used as flushing solutions.

Most angiographers use heparinized saline with heparin concentrations apparently ranging in different centres from 1 to 10 IU/ml. No study appears to exist to support the use of heparinization in this way, though it does not, of course, appear at all unreasonable. Many authorities would recommend the systemic heparinization of the patient for angioplasty procedures but there is no consensus on this either, except perhaps in the context of coronary angioplasty, and no controlled study has been carried out to demonstrate its efficacy.

It has been shown that, at least with multiple side hole and end hole catheters, the pressure of the flush is as important as the nature of the flushing solution. Low pressure flushes the side holes, and indeed sometimes only the more proximal side holes, and higher pressure is needed to flush the end hole and prevent clot formation here [3].

It is the author's belief that frequent and vigorous flushing is far more important than the precise nature of the flushing solution and is the critical point of good angiographic technique [3].

References

1. Dawson P et al (1986) Contrast, coagulation and fibrinolysis. Invest Radiol 21:248–252
2. Dawson P (1988) Non-ionic contrast agents and coagulation. Invest Radiol 23:310–317
3. Dawson P, Strickland NS (1991) Thromboembolic phenomena in clinical angiography: role of materials and technique. JVIR (in press)
4. Hawkins IF, Herbeth (1974) Contrast material used as a catheter flushing agent: a method to reduce clot formation during angiography. Radiology 110:351–352
5. Miller DL (1989) Heparin in angiography: current patterns of use. Radiology 172:1007–1011
6. Robertson HJF (1987) Blood clot formation in angiographic syringes containing non-ionic contrast media. Radiology 162:621–622

CHAPTER 8

Adverse Reactions and Their Pathophysiology and Management

8.1 What Adverse Reactions Can be Expected After Administration of Contrast Media?

R. Grainger

The ideal radiological contrast medium (RCM) should produce no adverse reaction (AR) and the patient should be unaware that he has received an injection, either intravenous or intraarterial. No RCM yet developed has achieved this ideal performance but with the low osmolar contrast media (LOCM) major gains have been made in this respect for both intravenous and intraarterial injection.

AR may be due to the hyperosmolality of the CM and are therefore concentration and dose dependent, or they may be of unknown cause – generally described as anaphylactoid because of a similarity to true anaphylactic reactions. These anaphylactoid reactions are neither clearly osmolar nor dose dependent and deaths have been recorded with test doses as small as 1 ml.

The time of onset of AR may be immediately during the injection but are usually delayed a few minutes. About 60% of early reactions begin within 5 min of the injection; another 30% begin within the next 10–20 min. The patient must therefore not be left unobserved, at least during this period.

Intravenous Injection

There is no general consensus as to what should be regarded as an AR. For example, a hot flush is a physiological consequence of the injection of a large volume of very high osmolar fluid, i.e. 50–100 ml high osmolar contrast media (HOCM) at 300 mg I/ml, which has five times the physiological osmolality.

These AR to intravenous injections are, however, not entirely dependent on osmolality, as ioxaglate (which has the lowest osmolality of current LOCM but which is ionic) produces more AR on intravenous injection than the nonionic LOCM, but fewer AR than ionic HOCM. It may well be that ionicity as well as osmolality is a factor in the production of AR (particularly nausea, vomiting, minor skin reactions) on intravenous injection.

Minor Reactions

The more frequent minor AR to RCM are, in descending order

1. Hot flush especially affecting the face, neck, external genitalia
2. Pruritis, minor hives or urticaria
3. Nausea, vomiting, disordered taste, sneezing
4. A general feeling of anxiety by the patient
5. Coughing and dyspnoea
6. Pain at the injection site sometimes projected proximally along the vein.

The incidence of these minor sensations is much more frequent (up to 10%–20%) with HOCM than with LOCM (2%–4%), depending on the volume, hypertonicity of the RCM, patient reactivity and anxiety, and whether a hot flush is regarded as an AR.

Many intravenous injections of LOCM cause no discomfort or AR and the patient may be unaware that an injection is being made.

Intermediate AR

Intermediate AR are more serious degrees of the symptoms mentioned above, especially urticaria, vomiting, dyspnoea and anxiety.

Bronchospasm with increasing dyspnoea and moderate hypotension may occur and the patient may feel apprehensive and anxious. The incidence of these intermediate reactions is about 0.5%–1.00% for HOCM and probably 25% this incidence for LOCM.

Severe AR

Severe AR are usually severe manifestations of the above-mentioned minor and intermediate reactions, especially dyspnoea, bronchospasm, hypotension, severe apprehension sometimes accompanied by uncontrolled restlessness, angioneurotic oedema of the glottis, one or more grand mal convulsions and disturbed consciousness. Bronchospasm may become severe and the airway may be threatened by severe laryngeal and neck oedema. Cardiovascular collapse may develop suddenly with pulmonary oedema, severe hypotension, shock with diminished cardiac venous return, cardiac arrhythmias and possibly cardiac arrest.

Full emergency cardiorespiratory resuscitation is imperative, demanding well-organized and rehearsed procedures with immediate access to a crash trolley complete with DC defibrillator and competent medical assistance, including an experienced anaesthetist. The incidence of these severe reactions is up to 0.2% for HOCM injections and up to 0.04% for LOCM injections.

Death

In a few patients the severe AR may become extreme and may not respond even to the most energetic, expert and immediate resuscitation. The most common causes of death are cardiorespiratory collapse, pulmonary oedema, deepening coma, intractable bronchospasm and airway obstruction.

In a very few patients, sudden death may occur shortly after the injection, presumably from cardiovascular shock and arrhythmia but without prodromal symptoms.

The mortality rate from intravenous RCM injections is not known with any degree of precision and retrospective analyses of large series provide mortality rates ranging from 1 in 15,000 to 1 in 170,000 intravenous injections of HOCM. A mortality range of 1 in 40,000 to 1 in 80,000 is likely. It is uncertain whether this rate will be significantly reduced with LOCM injections, but it seems likely that the mortality rate may be reduced by a factor of two or more with injection of these new products.

Intra-arterial Injections

All of the above AR may occur following intra-arterial injection. The incidence is lower by perhaps a factor of two or three, compared with intravenous injection of the same product.

Peripheral arterial injection (carotid, vertebral or limb arteries) of RCM at osmolalities above 600 mOsm/kg water invariably cause a hot flush sometimes with severe pain in the injected arterial territory. This feature is definitely osmolar dependent and is greatly reduced in frequency and in severity when diluted HOCM (for digital imaging) or LOCM are injected. Injections of RCM into the aorta may cause substantial flushing, headache, vasodilatation and hypotension which are much more frequent and severe with HOCM compared to LOCM injections. Pulmonary artery injections may cause coughing, chest discomfort and dyspnoea, again more severe with HOCM injections. Visceral injections either with HOCM or LOCM do not usually cause discomfort.

It is advisable that the patient be forewarned of any likely discomfort following RCM injection and he should be reassured that the symptoms, although uncomfortable, are temporary and rarely require treatment.

8.2 Do Late-Occurring Adverse Reactions to Contrast Media Necessitate Longer Supervision of the Patient?

P. Davies

Definition of Delayed (Late-Occurring) Adverse Reactions

Delayed reactions have been defined as those that occur after the patient has left the department [3]. The time spent in the department after the injection is rather variable. Further, there are several types of delayed reactions:
1. Venous problems – thrombosis and skin necrosis;
2. rashes;
3. a "flu-like syndrome";
4. parotitis;
5. cardiac syndromes – worsening of heart failure and cardiac arrest.

Time of Onset of Acute Reactions

Acute reactions are clearly those that occur while the patient is under observation in the department.

Acute deaths and severe life-threatening reactions with ionic (high osmolar) agents occur early, most within 15 min but about 10% occur after this time, some later than 60 min [6].

About two-thirds of such reactions occur within 5 min of injection [6] so that observation of the patient is most important early on. It is the author's practice when performing a urography to stay in the examination room talking to the patient until asked by the radiographer to inspect the 5-min film (about 7 min) which makes a natural break. After a brief inspection to check on the compression band (if used) further observation is left to the radiographers.

Some patients may suffer a cardiac arrest. This is an event which may occur at any time. The difficulty in such cases is to determine whether it could truly be attributed to the injection and some cases have been reported before an injection was made [4].

Are Delayed Reactions Serious or Fatal

In none of the studies from Nottingham were delayed deaths reported and the author is not aware of any studies indicating that delayed life-threatening reactions occur.

In the Bristol study [1] the most important serious reaction was worsening or onset of heart failure in patients recovering from heart attacks. It has been noted that deaths in patients suffering from cardiac disease tend to be delayed beyond 5 min [4]; after an hour it is difficult to be sure the death is due to the contrast medium [4].

Some patients suffer a constitutional illness which they certainly regard as serious enough to confine them to bed.

With high-osmolar agents, late skin necrosis requiring skin grafting occurred sometimes after extravasation of CM beneath the skin, although usually there are no sequelae. Unlike acute rashes the delayed rashes appear to be reproducible on challenge but no large study has been done to test this observation. When it recurs the rash is the same as it was on the previous occasion. Acute rashes do not predict delayed rashes and in any case only affect one-third of cases on challenge [5].

Heart failure may be avoided by not examining patients who have suffered a myocardial infarction until they are fully recovered from the cardiovascular instability. Previous heart disease was not found to be a risk factor in the Nottingham study [2].

Conclusion

Careful selection of patients for CM studies is important. Late reactions cannot be predicted or avoided by observation and continuous observation to detect acute serious reactions is most important in the first 5 min after injection.

References

1. Davies P, Roberts MB, Roylance J (1975) Acute reactions to urographic contrast media. BMJ 1:434–437

2. McCullogh M, Davies P, Richardson RE (1989) A large trial of intravenous Conray 325 and Niopam 300 to assess immediate and delayed reaction. Br Radiol 62:260–265
3. Panto P, Davies P (1986) Delayed reactions to urographic contrast media. Br J Radiol 59:41–44
4. Pendergrass HP, Tondreau RL, Pendergrass EP, Ritchie DJ, Hildreth EA, Askovitz SI (1958) Reactions associated with intravenous urography: historical and statistical review. Radiology 71:1–12
5. Witten DM, Hirsch FD, Hartman GW (1973) Acute reactions to urographic contrast medium. AJR 119:832–840
6. Wolfram R, Dehouve A, Degand F, Wattez E, Lange R, Crehalet A (1965) Les accidents graves par injection intraveineuse de substances iodées pour urographie. J Electrologie 47:346–357

8.3 Do Late Reactions Occur More Frequently After Administration of Non-ionic Contrast Media?

P. Davies

The null hypothesis is that there is no difference in the frequency of late reactions between ionic and nonionic media and this must be disproved in order to demonstrate greater safety of one or the other.

Venous problems are certainly lessened by the use of low osmolar agents but about 10% of patients report arm pain after an injection of a low osmolar medium [2].

Heart failure should be less frequent because of the lowered osmolality but no study has shown this and some cardiac problems occur when no injection has been made [3].

There is less pain after extravasation and so skin necrosis should occur less frequently.

Rashes and parotitis were reported by McCullough, Davies and Richardson [2] to be more common with a nonionic agent. This seemed inherently unlikely and when more cases had been studied the combined results (reported by Davies at the ICR Paris [1] showed that there was no statistically significant difference in the incidence of rashes between the two groups of CM. Parotitis may, however, be more common with low osmolar media. Thus some reactions are reduced, others have the same incidence for the two groups of CM and very large numbers in controlled trials are required to answer the more interesting questions [2].

References

1. Davies P (1989) Abstracts of the International Congress of Radiology, Paris. Abstract 2173, p 344
2. McCullogh M, Davies P, Richardson RE (1989) A large trial of intravenous Conray 325 and Niopam 300 to assess immediate and delayed reactions. Br J Radiol 62:260–265
3. Pendergrass HP, Tondreau RL, Pendergrass EP, Ritchie DJ, Hildreth EA, Askovitz SI (1958) Reactions associated with intravenous urography: historical and statistical review. Radiology 71:1–12

8.4 What Are the Mediators of Anaphylactoid Reactions to Iodinated Contrast Media?

P. Dawson

The mechanisms of major anaphylactoid reactions to iodinated CM remain unclear. The consensus emerging is that classical anaphylaxis involving IgE antibodies is not involved, though see Sects 8.7 and 8.8.

CM are known to be capable of activation of the complement system, though by which pathway is uncertain. The role of this in major reactions is certainly not established and in some studies appears to occur rather routinely both in vitro and in vivo.

Histamine has long been considered the major mediator in CM major reactions. It can be released from mast cells by direct, nonimmunological mechanisms. CM are certainly capable of this but the problem is that such release of histamine can be found, once again, routinely in patients receiving contrast and not at significantly higher levels in patients experiencing major reactions. However, it is difficult to dismiss the idea of a role for histamine since it is capable of producing at least four of the major abnormalities which characterize severe reactions, namely bronchospasm, oedema, urticaria and hypotension.

Bradykinin may elicit the same responses as histamine but is considerably more potent on a molar basis than is histamine. Elevation of plasma bradykinin levels has been noted following CM injection clinically. The production of bradykinin involves a complex sequence of proteolytic events beginning with the activation of factor XII, which is, incidentally, the initiating part of the coagulation/contact system. This initiation may take place because of endothelial injury by CM (more marked with high osmolality agents) or, perhaps, by direct contact activation by the agents themselves.

Another intriguing fact concerning bradykinin is that it can also produce mobilization of arachidonic acid and thus provide the basis for the production of leucotrienes and prostaglandins. These are, indeed, widely held to play at least some role in anaphylactic and anaphylactoid reactions generally.

One clinical study in the context of intravenous injections demonstrated no significant increase in the levels of leucotrience C4 but other studies, with a variety of CM, have demonstrated significant increases in PGI2 thromboxane A_2 but no change in thromboxane B_2. These observations certainly suggest that some CM are capable of stimulating vascular endothelium, and perhaps white cells, to release prostacyclin.

It must be stressed that too little work has been done in this area because of its difficulty and that the individual and joint roles of various mediators cannot yet be dogmatically stated.

8.5 What Adverse Reactions to Contrast Media Are Dose Independent or Dependent?

H. Katayama

Adverse reactions can be divided into two categories: physicochemotoxic and idiosyncratic reactions [3]. The physicochemical reactions are directly related to dose and are primarily due to the hypertonicity and viscosity of the CM.

Idiosyncratic reactions are not considered to be dose related and can occur with so-called small doses of 1 ml or less of CM. Clinical symptoms are shown in Table 8.5.1.

It has been claimed that the incidence of reactions with infusion pyelography is no greater or less than that with conventional pyelography. The results from Ansell's [1, 2] survey do not support this claim. The incidence of reactions appears to be at least three times greater with infusion pyelography. According to Ansell [1, 2], taking a dividing line

Table 8.5.1. Clinical symptoms of adverse reactions to CM

physicochemotoxic reaction (dose related)	Idiosyncratic reaction (not dose related)
Heat sensation	Life-threatening or fatal reaction
Vascular pain	Severe hypotension
Hypervolemia	Loss of consciousness
Endothelial injury	Convulsion
Erythrocyte damage	Pulmonary oedema
Decreased renal function	Urticaria
Arrythmia	Larnygeal oedema
Paralysis and convulsion	Bronchospasm
Coagulation deficit	Cardiac arrest

at 20 g of iodine, there were fewer cases of severe reactions below this level. Most of them were in patients with a history of cardiac disease or allergy.

However, according to Katayama's survey [4], for ionic CM the prevalence of adverse reactions was lower in the subgroup receiving more than 80 ml; for nonionic CM, the prevalence was lowest in the

Table 8.5.2. Prevalence of adverse drug reactions by dose (from [4])

Dose (ml)	Cases with ionic CM		Cases with nonionic CM	
	Total (*n*)	ADR (*n*) (%)	Total (*n*)	ADR (*n*) (%)
<20	4139	916 (22,13)	8401	334 (3,98)
21–40	17286	3235 (18,71)	13585	652 (4,80)
41–60	11135	1824 (16,38)	7940	411 (5,18)
61–80	3684	736 (19,98)	4994	247 (4,95)
81–100	103231	11681 (11,32)	120792	3024 (2,50)
>101	29488	2920 (9,90)	12344	564 (4,57)
No entry	321	... ...	307	... ...

ADR, adverse drug reactions

subgroup receiving 81–100 ml (Table 8.5.2). There is general agreement that there are dose-related or -dependent adverse reactions, but injection rates are factors which clearly bear on the incidence of adverse reactions. Dose of contrast media and rate of injection should be considered together.

References

1. Ansell G et al (1980) The current status of reactions to i. v. CM. Invest Radiol [Suppl]:32–39
2. Ansell G (1970) Adverse reactions to CA. Invest Radiol 6:374–384
3. Committee on Drugs of the American College of Radiology (1977) Prevention and management of adverse reactions to intravascular contrast media. American College of Radiology, Chicago, pp 1–3
4. Katayama H et al (1990) Adverse reaction to ionic and non-ionic CM. Radiology 175:621–628

8.6 Are Antibodies to Radiographic Contrast Media Known?

R. C. Brasch

Allergy is one of the mechanisms proposed for CM toxicity. This theory incorporates the assumption that antibodies reactive with CM molecules exist in humans either as naturally occurring antibodies or as antibodies induced by prior exposure to CM itself or by exposure to structurally similar molecules. It is possible and precedented for atopic individuals to produce antibodies, induced by one chemical, that cross-react with another chemical; for example, antibodies induced by penicillin may also produce an allergic reaction to cephalosporins.

There can be little doubt that antibodies reactive to CM exist in humans. Harboe et al. in 1976 observed sudden death in a patient caused by interaction between an IgM antibody and ioglycamide [3]. In this startling case the antibody was a paraprotein, present in very high concentration, and upon injection of the CM a gelatinous precipitate formed in the antecubital vein, right heart and pulmonary vessels. Subsequently, Bauer reported on the extensive immunological characterization of this anti-CM antibody [1].

Additional patients suffering severe CM reactions with demonstration of antibody activity towards the offending agent were reported by Kleinknecht et al. [4] (iothalamate induction of dyspnoea, bronchospasm, pulmonary oedema, and renal failure) and by Wakkers-Garritsen and co-workers [5] (dyspnoea, circulatory collapse, and unconsciousness). Adding to the evidence for existence of antibodies to CM is the report from our laboratory showing that antibody binding activity (Farr radioimmunoassay system) in the sera from 27 reacting patients was significantly elevated as compared to assay results from non-reacting control patients [2].

For the present, critical unanswered questions are
1. what proportion of all patients suffering severe CM reactions have anti-CM antibodies, and

2. what is the optimal assay system to detect these potentially reacting patients?

References

1. Bauer K (1978) Antigen-antibody like reaction of ioglycamide with an IgM paraprotein in vivo and in vitro. In: Zeitler E (Hrsg.) Neue Aspekte des Kontrastmittel-Zwischenfalls. Schering, Berlin, pp 71–78
2. Brasch RC, Caldwell JL (1976) The alergic theory of radiocontrast agent toxicity: demonstration of antibody activity in sera of patients suffering major radiocontrast agent reactions. Invest Radiol 11:347–356
3. Harboe M, Folling I, Haugen OA, Bauer K (1976) Sudden death caused by interaction between a macroglobulin and a divalent drug. Lancet 79/80:285–288
4. Kleinknecht D, Deloux J, Homberg JC (1974) Acute renal failure after intravenous urography: detection of antibodies against contrast media: Clin Nephrol 2:116
5. Wakkers-Garritsen BG, Houwerziji J, Nater JP, Wakkers PJM (1976) IgE-mediated adverse reactivity to a radiographic contrast medium-case report. Ann Allergy 36:122

8.7 Are There Allergies to Contrast Media?

R. C. Brasch

A considerable body of evidence has been accumulated indicating that certain patients suffer immediate antibody-mediated adverse drug reactions (ADR) to iodinated CM. ADRs clinically resemble known allergic symptoms, including urticaria, bronchospasm, laryngeal oedema, facial swelling and circulatory collapse. Virtually every large epidemiological study has shown an unusually high incidence of CM reactions among allergic individuals, particularly asthmatics. Further supporting the allergic hypothesis is the fact that antibodies (IgG and IgE) have been successfully induced in rabbits [2] and guinea pigs [1] using CM bound to carrier proteins. Further, the degree of spontaneous protein binding observed with different CM correlates directly with the rate of ADRs. Guinea pigs, in which anti-CM antibodies have been induced, have been shown to suffer anaphylactic death when challenged with iodinated CM [1]. In Sect. 8.6 specific case histories were described of patients with severe reactions in whom specific anti-CM antibodies were demonstrated. These antibodies may occur naturally (without prior exposure to the specific allergen) or may be induced by exposure to CM themselves or to structurally similar molecules. We have all had contact with halogenated benzene rings (like CM) and such exposure in atopic individuals may induce antibody formation.

Current scientific challenges include the development of highly sensitive and specific immunoassays for anti-CM antibodies. These may permit identification of the allergic individual prior to exposure or may indicate which of several CM could be administered safely without antibody reactivity. Not all ADRs to CM need to be on an allergic basis; differing mechanisms may be operative in different patients.

References

1. Brasch RC (1980) Evidence supporting an antibody mediation of contrast media reactions. Invest Radiol 15 [Suppl]:S29–S31
2. Brasch RC, Caldwell JL, Fudenberg HH (1976) Antibodies to radiographic contrast agents: induction and characterization of rabbit antibody. Invest Radiol 11:1–9

8.8 Can Sensitization Due to Frequent Contrast Media Administration Be Observed?

R. C. Brasch

Generally, the large epidemiological studies of adverse drug reactions (ADR) to iodinated CM have shown no increase in the reaction rates for patients with previous exposure to CM. Sandstrom [2] reported his experience with over 7000 patients, some of whom had as many as seven previous CM studies and noted no relationship between number of exposures and rate of reactions. More recently, Katayama et al. [1] reported on observations in 337 647 patients receiving either ionic or low-osmolar nonionic CM; rates for ADRs were significantly lower using the nonionic CM. However, there was no increase in reactivity among the patients with prior CM exposure (6.9%) when compared to patients with no history of prior CM administration (8.6%). Of course, these epidemiological reports do not totally exclude the possibility that a given patient may be sensitized by CM. It should be noted that CM have a relatively short residence time within the body due to their rapid elimination by glomerular filtration, thereby precluding the lengthy exposure that may be required to induce an immunological response. As mentioned earlier, patients may be sensitized by prior exposure to chemicals structurally similar to CM, any halogenated benzene ring for instance and antibodies so induced may cross-react when CM is administered.

References

1. Katayama H, Yamaguchi K, Kosuka T, Takashima T, Seez P, Matsuura K (1990) Adverse reactions to ionic and nonionic contrast media. A report from the Japanese Committee on the Safety of contrast Media. Radiology 175:621–628
2. Sandstrom C (1955) Secondary reactions from contrast media and the allergy concept. Acta Radiol [Diagn] (Stockh) 44:233

8.9 Can Epileptogenicity and Arachnoiditis Be Observed After Myelography with Nonionic Contrast Media?

I. O. Skalpe

Compared with ionic CM the epileptogenicity and frequency of postmyelographic arachnoiditis with metrizamide (Amipaque) were very low. With the introduction of iohexol (Omnipaque) these problems seem to be virtually eliminated. Thus, we have not seen any epileptic seizure nor any case of postmyelographic arachnoiditis during our more than 6 years of experience with iohexol myelography, comprising more than 1500 examinations.

8.10 Are Contrast Media Dialysable?

J. E. Scherberich

CM can normally be well dialysed. The dialysability of conventional CM is about 55 ml/min in a blood flow of ca. 200ml/min, when dialysers with cupreous membranes are used. However, in chronic dialysis patients, significant CM concentrations are still measurable in the blood 7 days after administration, in spite of further regular haemodialysis; this results from the redistribution of CM to the extravascular space. If CM are administered to patients undergoing chronic haemodialysis in diagnostic or therapeutic examinations, this must occur either before a planned dialysis treatment or be followed by dialysis within 3 h.

CHAPTER 9

Clinical Use of Iodinated Contrast Media for the Visualization of Vessels, Organs and Organ Systems

9.1 Carotid and Vertebral Arteries and Cerebral Vessels

I. O. Skalpe

Following the introduction of a series of noninvasive imaging modalities (CT, MRI, Doppler sonography) during the last two decades the indications for cerebral angiography have been markedly reduced and consequently the number of examinations has been dramatically diminished, in most centers by more than 50%. Thus, angiography is usually not indicated in head trauma, or in brain tumours, both of which were important indications for cerebral angiography prior to the CT era. One may expect this trend to continue, since MRI angiography will reduce the need for conventional cerebral angiography even further.

The most important indications for cerebral angiography today are diseases in the cerebral vessel:
a) Degenerative lesions (arteriosclerosis)
b) arteritis
c) aneurysms and
d) arteriovenous malformations.

These indications will hold for the foreseeable future. One reason for this is the remarkable progress in endovascular treatment of these lesions in recent years.

Technique

The examination is usually performed via the transfemoral route under local anaesthesia. Following puncture of the femoral artery and introduction of the guide wire a preshaped catheter is introduced. Selective injections are then performed in both carotid arteries and in the left vertebral artery. We always start the examination with angiography of the aortic arch in patients with arteriosclerosis. A pigtail catheter is placed with the tip proximal to the brachiocephalic artery in these patients.

In conventional angiography using a cut-film changer the dose of CM is 8–10 ml (300 mg I/ml) in the carotids, 6 ml (300 mg I/ml) in the vertebral artery and 60 ml (350 mg I/ml) in the aortic arch. The injections are performed with a pressure injector. In intra-arterial digital subtraction angiography (IA-DSA) the dose per injection may be markedly reduced. However, since biplane exposure is not available in these systems, the number of injections must be increased. Thus, the total amount of CM in grams of iodine will be about the same.

The examination is usually easy to perform and may be completed within half an hour. Selective injections may be a problem in arteriosclerotic patients. Direct puncture and catheterization of the common carotid artery can be performed in these cases. In our department direct puncture is performed once or twice a year, whereas some centres use this approach routinely. The transaxillary or transbrachial route is used only in exceptional cases, since these carry a higher risk for local complications than the other methods.

Complications

In our opinion most complications in cerebral angiography are related more to the examination technique than to toxic effects of the CM. In a study of more than 2500 cerebral angiographies we found that there was no relationship between the occurrence of complications and
1. the number of CM injections per artery
2. the maximum amount of CM to one artery
3. the total amount of CM injected. More than one third of the complications were totally unpredictable, occurring after short-lasting examinations with no technical problems.

The most frequent complications in cerebral angiography are hemiparesis, dysarthria, visual disturbances and disturbances of consciousness. These are seen in 1%–2% of patients. In the majority the disturbances are transient with full recovery within 24 h. Permanent sequelae are extremely rare – 0.2% in the material mentioned above.

We believe that the majority of these complications are caused by embolism. During the catheterization procedure embolic material may be detached from arteriosclerotic lesions of the intima. Thrombus may form on the catheter wall and also within the catheter lumen and in the syringes where aspirated blood may come in conctact with the syringe wall. Such complications can, to some extent, be prevented by a meticulous technique. Thus, aspiration of blood into syringes should be avoided. This is even more important with nonionic than with ionic CM, since ionic CM have a stronger anticoagulant effect than nonionic CM. Furthermore, recent reports have shown that nonionic CM in mixture with blood generates thrombin, whereas this is not seen with ionic CM. It has been suggested on the basis of these in vitro experiments that nonionic CM may cause thromboembolism more often than ionic ones. This has not been our experience. We have used iohexol (Omnipaque) routinely for cerebral angiography for the last 7 years and compared with our previous experience with the ionic CM metrizoate (Isopaque Cerebral) there has been a minor reduction of the complication rate from 2% to 1.3%.

The following precautions are recommended when using nonionic CM in angiography: frequent flushing of the catheter with heparinized saline and minimal aspiration of blood into the syringes. Syringes should be plastic rather than glass, since in vitro experiments have demonstrated greater and faster thrombin generation in glass syringes than in plastic ones. Aspirin, which effectively reduces platelet aggregation, should be given 1–2 h prior to the examination. Following these guidelines, the full advantage of the definitely better biocompatibility of nonionic CM is obtained.

Although ionic CM are well tolerated in cerebral angiography with only minor complaints from the patients following injections into the cerebral arteries, these side effects are even less with nonionic CM. This is of practical importance in selective injections into the external carotid artery, where ionic CM often cause considerable pain and unpleasant warmth, whereas nonionics usually induce no unpleasant effects at all.

Local complications at the puncture site are very rare. Haematomas may occasionally occur, but are very rarely of clinical significance. Thrombosis of the femoral artery with total obliteration of the lumen has been reported, but this is extremely rare. However, it is important for the clinician to be aware of these possibilities, so that proper treatment can be instituted before irreversible damage ensues.

In conclusion, although ionic CM are relatively well tolerated in cerebral angiography, we recommend nonionic CM for this examination.

References

Fareed J, Walenga J, Saravia GE, Moncada RM (1990) Thrombogenic potential of nonionic contrast media? Radiology 174:321–325

Skalpe IO (1988) Complications in cerebral angiography with iohexol (Omnipaque) and meglumine metrizoate (Isopaque Cerebral). Neuroradiology 30:69–72

Skalpe IO, Nakstad P (1988) Myelography with iohexol (Omnipaque): a clinical report with special reference to the adverse effects. Neuroradiology 30:169–174

Skalpe IO, Sortland O (1989) Myelography. Lumbar-thoracic-cervical with water-soluble contrast medium. Textbook and atlas 2nd edn. Tano, Oslo

Stormorken H, Skalpe IO, Testart MC (1986) Effect of various contrast media on coagulation, fibrinolysis, and platelet function. An in vitro and in vivo study. Invest Radiol 21:348–354

9.2 Spinal Angiography and Phlebography

A. Thron

Spinal Angiography

Why?

The visualization of the blood vessels supplying the spinal canal, spinal cord, and cauda equina is presently only possible by means of selective angiography, since, due to the smallness of the structures (anterior spinal artery < 1 mm), a high degree of spatial and contrast resolution is required. Noninvasive procedures such as US or MRI do not yield comparable images. Even with flush aortography, the branch vessels from the segmental arteries to the axial skeleton, and especially to the spinal canal, cannot be adequately demonstrated. For this reason, selective study of the segmental arteries branching off from the aortic arch or of their homologues is the method of choice. Before the introduction of digital subtraction angiography (DSA), the photographic film subtraction of standard cut-film angiography was required to eliminate overlapping by bony structures. This procedure was not only very time-consuming and expensive, but was also diagnostically unsatisfactory, since, frequently, diagnostic assessment was not possible until the film subtractions were available. Given that a complete selective spinal angiography requires serial angiograms of 30–35 individual arteries, it is easy to see what an advance the introduction of DSA represented. It makes a substracted image – with somewhat less spatial resolution but higher contrast resolution – and thus diagnostic information immediately available. The advantageous contrast resolution enables the injection of less concentrated CM solutions. Combined with the obligatory use of nonionic CM which are less neurotoxic and less damaging to vascular endothelium, the previously much feared spinal angiography has become a safe examination procedure.

When?

Spinal angiography is indicated in the following situations: suspected spinal vascular malformation (AV malformation, cavernoma); suspected spinal dural AV fistula; preoperatively, in tumours of the spinal cord or spinal column; and preoperatively, preceding scoliosis operations.

The clinically tentative diagnosis of a spinal infarct generally does not represent an indication. This diagnosis first has to be deduced from: the clinical picture (acute transverse lesion with zonal pain), an unhelpful result of other imaging procedures (myelography, MRI), an unimpressive analysis and, if applicable, anamnestic signs (embolizing heart disease, condition following aortic surgery, dissecting aortic aneurysm). It is almost impossible practically to prove that a spinal infarct results from the occlusion of an artery supplying the spinal cord. This is due to the great variability in the arteries supplying the spinal cord and to their small calibre, which only allow inconstant and segmental visualization. Even if a vascular occlusion were proven, this would still not have specific therapeutic consequences. Often the diagnosis can be corroborated by MRI follow-up examinations.

An indication can, however, arise if, in a subacute presentation, the findings of myelographic or MRI examination raise the question of a differential diagnostis of a spinal vascular malformation. It is difficult to say whether spinal angiography in search of a spinal vascular malformation or a dural AV fistula is indicated in progressive, clinical, transverse spinal cord syndrome even without such findings. As a rule, the suspected clinical condition should be corroborated through evidence of conspicuous dilated vessels in the subarachnoid space. In spinal AV dural fistula with localization of the "angioma" in the dura mater spinalis and drainage of the shunt via superficial veins of the spinal cord, this vascular dilatation can be very inconspicuous. As so-called varicosis spinalis, this finding can often be better recognized on a technically well-performed myelogram than in MRI. However, the latter provides better evidence of central inner medullary spinal cord damage over long segments resulting from excessive pressure and volume strain on the spinal venous system. In this way, it may also be a diagnostic indicator.

Tumours of the spinal cord or spinal column are a relative indication for angiography. Such a procedure should provide the operator with information about spinal feeders in the neighbourhood of the space-occupying lesion and allow him to make an assessment of the degree of vascularity and of the possibility of its preoperative embolization. Before a severe scoliosis is straightened, the entry levels of the vessels supplying the spinal cord should also be known in order to avoid damaging them.

Premises

1. Selective spinal angiography should only be performed, if at all possible, at centres specializing in it and possessing sufficient experience. Facilities for DSA have to be considered practically obligatory today. The operator has to be well-acquainted with spinal vascular anatomy and possess enough information to confirm there is a good indication.
2. From the patient's view point, the same premises hold for spinal angiography that hold for other examinations involving the administration of iodinated X-ray CM or for other angiographies requiring transfemoral entry (see Chap. 9.3).

How?

Selective spinal angiography can practically only be performed via the trans-femoral route. If this path of entry is impossible, only diagnostically inade-quate survey angiography or individual-vessel studies in the cervical region are possible via a transbrachial or axillary procedure.

After puncture of the inguinal artery, a catheter sheath should always be used, since the changing directions in which the segmental arteries branch off along the course of the aorta may make it necessary to change the catheter repeatedly. The catheter used has to display a curvature of its tip; on the one hand, it has to be adjusted to the changing lumen width of the aorta, and on the other it has to permit the catheter tip to slip into the ostia of the intercostal or lumbar arteries. If the catheters are not shaped by the examiner himself, he has to have several potentially suitable tip curvatures at his disposal. The order in which the ostia of the lumbar and intercostal arteries are probed is unimportant. However, it is advisable to maintain an examination protocol in which it is noted which vessels have already been visualized. A metal marker projected paravertebrally on the patient's back facilitates rapid determination of the catheter level. The catheter tip should not occlude the ostium and if aspiration of blood is difficult in small vessels, one has to be careful to keep the catheter connection free of air.

For visualization of individual segmental arteries, 1–2 ml nonionic CM are injected, using the DSA technique, in a concentration of 200 mg I/ml and in a standard cut-film technique in a concentration of 300 mg I/ml. In the case of the confirmation of an AV malformation, selective angiography can be performed, depending on shunt volume, with 5 ml CM (in exceptional cases more) in the above-mentioned concentrations. A series of pictures taken laterally should then be made, something that can be omitted in the event of normal findings. The length of an angiographic series, even in the search for vascular malformations, should not be less than 4–5 s. The exploration of the supra-aortic arteries (vertebral artery, costocervical trunk and thyrocer-vical trank) requires a less curved universal or headhunter catheter. An injection dose of 4–5 ml CM (200–250 mg I/ml) is required for the vertebral artery. Since no more than a total of 300 ml nonionic CM (at a concentration of 300 mg I/ml) should be administered, in rare cases involving older pa-tients, a second session might be required for a complete spinal angiogra-phy. The preoperative visualization of the vascular supply of a spinal tumour can be limited to the corresponding region of the spinal column; however, in tumours located in the spinal cord (e. g., haemangioblastoma), the radicular arteries merging into the spinal artery, above and below the tumour should also always be included.

In the search for the feeders of an AV malformation in the spinal cord or subarachnoid space, complete spinal angiography is necessary due to the frequency of multiple feeders. In spinal AV dura fistula, a complete thora-columbar study is desirable. In case this creates problems in the often older patients, a more limited study may also suffice if the shunt-feeding vessel is detected. One should under no circumstances hold spinal angiography to be negative if the search for a suspected spinal vascular malformation was not complete because some segmental arteries were omitted! A complete spinal angiography requires the visualization of both sides of the iliolumbar artery, the lumbar arteries, the intercostal arteries, the costocervical trunk, the thyrocervical trunk, and the vertebral artery. If there are no AV shunts, a visualization of the medullary-surface veins, directly responsible for draining the spinal cord, cannot be expected with the CM amounts given above.

Complications I: Those Induced by the Method

The potential complications related to the technical procedure correspond generally to those that can occur when the same procedure is applied to angiography of other vascular regions (see for example, Sect 9.3 "Angiography of the Extremities").

In order to avoid injuring the vascular wall with a catheter with marked tip curvature, a soft guidewire protruding in front of the tip should be used for the passage through the pelvic arteries. Injuries to the vascular wall at the ostia of the segmental arteries can lead to circumscribed dissections with or without the occurrence of spasm; they are almost always free of sequelae if the problem is immediately recognized and the catheter is removed. Due to the numerous, rope-ladder-like, extraspinal collaterals, the vascular supply to the spinal cord is as a rule maintained even in the case of a complete obstruction of passage of a segmental artery. This is the case as long as the lumen obstruction does not extend all the way to the point where a radicular artery that supplies the spinal cord exits from the obstructed artery. Thus, the correct positioning of the catheter tip and a careful catheter injection with obviously free CM flow are clearly necessary if spinal cord damage is to be avoided. All other potential complications (secondary bleeding, iatrogenic AV fistula, fever, nerve damage) are to be avoided or treated according to the instructions found in the section on angiography of the extremities.

Complications II: Those Induced by the Iodinated Contrast Medium

The following complications can be induced by the iodinated CM:
1. Hypersensitivity reaction up to anaphylactoid shock (see Sects. 8.1, 8.3, 8.4)
2. Cardiovascular reaction (see Sects. 3.4, 4.6)
3. Disturbance of kidney function (see Sects. 3.7, 4.8)
4. Coagulation disorders (see Sect. 3.3)
5. Damage to the intima or endothelium (see Sects. 3.11)
6. Neurological symptoms of irritation and disturbed function such as cortical blindness, myoclonus, and signs of partial to complete paraplegia.

The cause of specific neurological disorders may vary greatly. Clinically, one can hardly distinguish between vascular occlusion due to embolic material or coagulation disorders and toxic effects on vessels due to the CM used. Neurological deficits can be transient with full recovery or may result in a lasting deficit.

If symptoms of spinal irritation become manifest (electrical tingling in the extremities, myoclonus) all further CM injections must be avoided, unless these symptoms involve already existing spinal symptom from spinal injury.

Direct CM-induced organ damage to the spinal cord has been a problem to be taken seriously in both intentional and unintentional studies of the spinal arteries. CM myelopathy, formerly the model of an intermedullary microcirculatory disturbance, is in my own experience avoidable, if the above examination technique is used, and nonionic CM with little damaging effect on the endothelium and of low neurotoxicity are employed.

Conclusions

Selective spinal angiography using a DSA technique is the method of choice for visualizing AV malformations in the spinal canal; in cases where the latter is suspected, it absolutely must be used. Only by its use can the precise location of the AV shunt be determined, and the possibility and risks of treatment by surgery or embolization be assessed. Spinal angiography concomitant with operations on tumours of the spinal cord and vertebral column can also help improve the results of therapy. If the technique described here is followed and the obligatory use of nonionic CM accepted, previously feared complications can be reduced to such an extent that the approach to the case and discussions with the patient are associated with less anxiety.

Spinal Phlebography

Why?

Epidural venography practically stopped being utilized as a diagnostic procedure once CT and MRI allowed visualisation of even smaller, subtle space-occupying lesions in the neighbourhood of the spinal canal. Prior to this the procedure had been performed by a few specialists in order to recognize lateral disk prolapses, small extradural space-occupying lesions, or epidural angiomas that had escaped myelographic detection.

When?

Today the use of spinal phlebography can only rarely be justified and so little will be said about it here. This procedure may be indicated when, after all other diagnostic procedures (myelography, MRI, spinal arteriography) have been exhausted, the finding of a so-called varicosis spinalis with progressive symptoms of spinal disorder has remained uncertain. If, for corresponding circulatory disturbances of the spinal cord, an abnormal AV communication cannot be confirmed in the region of the dura mater spinalis, it would also be conceivable (though presently only hypothetically) that an obstruction of the drainage of the surface veins of the spinal cord into the epidural venous system might exist. In individual cases, this mechanism has been verified, when for example, due to agenesis of the inferior vena cava or other serious venous dysplasias, the epidural venous system has to take on the entire collateral drainage.

How?

The contrast visualization of the internal and external vertebral plexus of veins can be achieved through (a) intraosseous venography or (b) retrograde catheter venography. In the first case, the CM is injected into a spinous process of the vertebra or, in the neck region, into the cancellous bone of a vertebral body. In direct catheter venography using a transfemoral approach, the external and internal vertebral venous plexus can be visualized via the ascending lumbar veins in the lumbar region and by exploring the vertebral veins in the cervical region. In both cases, bilateral vascular catheterization with simultaneous CM injection is desirable, since in one-sided only injections, incomplete fillings all too frequently results, with a consequent danger of misinterpretation. Moreover, for the complete filling of the vertebral venous plexus over long stretches in the lower vertebral column segments, the inferior vena cava must be compressed using an inflatable rubber cuff. Injection pressure and volume depend on the catheter positioning.

Complications

These correspond to those in direct catheter venography in other regions.

Conclusion

Spinal phlebography is seldom used now in the routine diagnosis of vertebral and spinal space-occupying lesions. It is reserved for very specialized questions relating to circulatory disorders of spinal cord blood flow.

9.3 Angiography of the Extremities

H. J. Maurer

Why?

Angiography using a cut-film changer or 100-mm film remains the examination of highest spatial resolution, meaning that even very fine vessels (collaterals, tumour vessels) can be demonstrated. The format of the cut-film changer and the image intensifier allows the demonstration of larger vascular areas or of both lower extremities simultaneously. Although the spatial resolution of intra-arterial DSA is less, it allows the amounts of CM to be reduced; at the same time, however, the examination takes longer because of the need to readjust the equipment for each area to be investigated. Because the CM mixes with the venous blood, intravenous DSA provides poorer contrast and angiograms which are only partly free from overlap, particularly in the abdominal and retroperitoneal regions. In contrast to US, Doppler sonography and duplex sonography, angiography is relatively operator independent and reproducible. Another advantage of angiography is that the main examination can be followed by further selective studies and magnification techniques and, if necessary, by interventional procedures. Wherever possible, only nonionic iodinated preparations should be used as CM (see Chap. 3).

When?

Before angiography, an invasive procedure, is considered, alternative methods of noninvasive diagnosis should be exhausted:
– (Thermography)
– Doppler sonography
– Duplex sonography
– Colour sonography
– Plethysmography
– (MRI)

By demonstrating stenoses, occlusions, collateral circulations and suitable distal connector arteries, angiography will be able to make a major contribution to therapeutic decision making. The same applies to follow-up angiography after treatment, when functional investigations can also be performed; in this case, however, pretherapeutic measurements should be available so that comparisons can be made.

Preconditions

1. As with any examination with iodinated X-ray CM, the following information should be made available to the examiner: case history, clinical findings, results of any noninvasive vascular examinations, names of any drugs being taken at the time of the examination in view of possible interactions with the iodinated CM, any known allergies, previous hypersensitivity reactions – particularly to iodinated CM, clinical diagnosis and clinical question. Conclusions about the level of a stenosis or occlusion can be drawn beforehand from the level of the intermittent claudication.
2. The referring physician must ensure that no contraindication exists in respect of either the cardiovascular system, the kidneys or other organs. Thyroid diseases and paraproteinaemias weigh heavily in the consideration of benefits and risks; decisions should be taken after full discussion, as with patients with a known allergic case history or a previous reaction to CM.

Methods

Lower Extremities. The Seldinger technique permits (a) transfemoral or (b) transbrachial or transaxillary demonstration of both the abdominal aorta and the arteries of the pelvis and legs conventionally using cut-film, cine or intraarterial DSA. Intravenous DSA, the yield of which is clearly limited distal to the popliteal artery, may be performed in individual cases when vascular access is difficult and translumbar aortography (TLA) is not often necessary.

Upper Extremities. If the entire arm is to be demonstrated, it is advisable to use the transfemoral Seldinger technique with a preshaped catheter, the tip of which should be advanced beyond the origins of the extracranial cerebral vessels in order to prevent iodinated CM from entering the cerebral arteries. Direct antegrade or even retrograde puncture of the distal brachial artery is sufficient if only the distal lower arm and hand are to be demonstrated. In the shoulder – arm region, intravenous DSA leads to better results than in the demonstration of the arteries of the lower leg, but is hardly sufficient in the region of the hand because of the poorer contrast achieved. If transfemoral access is impossible, an approach may be made via the brachial artery on the opposite side with an appropriately preshaped catheter.

Procedure

One of the above-mentioned arteries is punctured under sterile conditions and an introducer is inserted through which the desired catheter is advanced. If necessary or desired, catheters can be changed without renewed trauma to the arterial wall.

The position of the pigtail catheter in aortoarteriography depends on the clinical question regarding the renal arteries. Because conventional angiography (cut-film changer) involves continuous, automatic moving of the patient, a test run is required to check the correct position; in cases of extreme bow legs or knock-knees, difficulties can arise in the region of the knees or distal lower leg. With the 100-mm film technique, the non- or only slightly absorbing sections between or around the limbs must be covered with Al filters or screened out by the equipment in both the conventional and the DSA procedures. Otherwise, the integrating dose measurement over the entire field would lead to underexposure. With DSA, readjustment must be performed for every vascular section to be investigated.

In the interest of reproducibility, the nonionic CM should always be injected with a high-pressure syringe. Up to 100 ml CM (300–370 mg I/ml) are administered for conventional aortoarteriography; the first film is obtained after a slight delay, the others according to predetermined data. Despite the five to seven adjustments required for intraarterial DSA, only about half of this amount of CM is required if no additional studies are necessary. The course of the pelvic arteries and the opening to the deep femoral artery may require additional adjustments, but not necessarily any particular increase of the amount of CM required. The same also applies to additional selective or superselective studies of arterial branches of interest after appropriate change of catheters.

If spasm occurs or is assumed, the examination should be repeated following an intra-arterial injection of a spasmolytic.

Angiography of the arm or distal lower arm and hand requires 10–20 ml of a nonionic CM (300–370 mg I/ml) and 5–10 ml, respectively, with both the conventional technique and intraarterial DSA.

Intravenous DSA, on the other hand, requires the injection of 40 ml of a nonionic CM (300–370 mg I/ml) for each run. The CM must be injected into the central venous system or left atrium under high pressure at a rate of 16–20 ml/s. Peripheral intravenous injection leads to (even) greater mixing with venous blood. An important problem with intravenous DSA is the transit time through the heart and pulmonary circulation, since it can make it very difficult – particularly in older patients with poor cardiac output and/or chronic pulmonary changes – to determine the time delay for the first film.

Wherever possible, no more than 300 ml nonionic contrast medium (300–370 mg I/ml) should be administered for angiography. This recommended value can be exceeded in the individual case depending on the cardiovascular system and the patient's condition. In such cases, however, careful monitoring is required for 24 h, and possibly 48 h, after angiography (see Sect. 3.7). If, despite everything, the lower leg arteries cannot be satisfactorily demonstrated in an individual case, intraoperative arteriography with puncture of the distal superficial femoral artery or popliteal artery can be undertaken.

Angiography of the arm or lower arm and hand always leads to good demonstration of the veins, something which cannot be achieved with aortoarteriography. If, however, filling of the venous system occurs in this region, then pathological conditions such as arteriovenous shunts are usually present.

Complications due to the Method

1. Haematomas of varying severity can occur on puncture of an artery or on introduction, of a venous line; this is the rule with direct aortography – the patient then often reports pain in the inguinal region. If the wall of the adjacent vein is injured during arterial puncture, an arteriovenous fistula requiring treatment may occasionally develop.
   If the case history indicates disturbance of blood clotting, great care must be taken to arrest the bleeding at the end of the examination and then to check on it afterwards.
2. If the material of venous lines, guidewires and catheters becomes defective or if the properties of disposable material change due to repeated use and sterilization, bending, fractures and breaks might occur and fragments may be washed away either into a peripheral artery or, in the case of intravenous DSA, into the heart or lungs and must then be removed.
3. Febrile reactions during and after angiography are not always attributable to the iodinated CM; other possibilities must also be checked wherever this is feasible, for example:
   a) inadequate resterilisation of disposable material;
   b) pyrogens in the CM ampoule or vial, even if they have not previously been demonstrated.
4. Malpositioning of the patient leading to injury to nerves, e. g. the ulnar nerve, must be avoided.
5. Piercing of a nerve on arterial puncture normally provokes an immediate reaction which, however, does not usually have any longer-lasting consequences. On the other hand, and although rare, extensive haematomas can lead to nerve compression or, in the axillary region, of the brachial plexus; close supervision is required in such cases so that countermeasures can be instituted in good time.
6. Atheromatous debris may become detached both on puncture and on introduction of venous lines, guidewires or catheters and may lead to peripheral embolism. Where applicable, the embolus must be removed.
7. In rare cases and despite careful introduction of the guidewire, the latter may pierce the arterial wall after undermining a plaque and either leave the wall again and return to the lumen or even remain in the wall. After the catheter has been advanced over the guidewire, this dissection may not be noticed during the test injection, meaning that the examination proceeds as planned and the error is not recognized until images or the

monitor is viewed; there are not usually any serious sequelae. In the other case, the CM runs off slowly and spreads like a dish in the arterial wall; again, serious sequelae follow only in occasional cases.

8. If the catheter tip is located under a plaque during the injection, the high pressure employed can cause varying amounts of the CM to enter the wall and, partly, to pass through it, to be demonstrated after the end of the examination as mural infiltration or extravascular contrast.

Complications due to the Iodinated Contrast Medium

1. Hypersensitivity reactions ranging up to anaphylactoid shock (see Sect. 4.1, 4.2)
2. Cardiovascular reaction (see Sect. 3.4)
3. Impairment of renal function (see Sect. 3.7, 4.8)
4. Clotting disturbances (see Sects. 2.15, 3.2, 3.3) and damage to intima or endothelium (see Sect. 3.11)
5. CNS reaction with occasional disturbance of vision ranging up to unilateral or bilateral amaurosis (see Sect. 3.10).

Wherever possible, a check should be made immediately to determine whether the event is a hypersensitivity, anaphylactoid reaction or a primary cardiovascular reaction, since the treatment to be instituted depends on this differentiation.

Apart from acute reactions, late reactions occurring up to 24 h after the examination are also known; reactions occurring even later have also been described in rare cases. In view of this, the patient should be closely observed after the end of the examination. Whereas there are no problems here as regards hospitalized patients, close collaboration with the referring doctor or hospital is required in the case of outpatient examinations.

For the management of acute reactions, the drugs and equipment required for appropriate therapy (i. e. defibrillator, intubation kit, needles and giving sets) must be readily available in the radiology department and, if possible, in the angiography room itself.

Outpatients who have undergone angiography must be observed for at least 2–3 h in the department or on a recovery ward before they are discharged to the care of the referring doctor or hospital.

If a moderately severe or severe reaction is observed in a radiological practice, it is advisable to transport the patient by ambulance to an intensive care unit.

The referring doctor or the doctor into whose care the patient has been placed must, of course, be given all available data both when the angiographic examination is without incident and, in particular, when a CM reaction occurs. Too little information can be fatal, particularly if a patient has had a previous CM reaction. If, despite all precautionary measures including previous prophylaxis (see Sects. 5.5, 5.6) and correct performance of the examination, a severe incident or one requiring treatment occurs, the examiner should take samples of venous and, if applicable, of arterial blood and of cerebrospinal fluid so that he can defend himself in the event of legal proceedings; a note should also be made of the batch number of the CM injected and any remaining CM saved. Since there are various reasons for a fatal outcome of a CM reaction, a forensic postmortem examination should always be requested in such cases.

Conclusion

Because the intravascular use of iodinated CM can provoke dose-dependent reactions, intraarterial DSA is now the method of choice for all angiographic examinations. Where the object is to visualize fine and extremely fine vessels, however, conventional film angiography should be performed. In a number of cases, intravenous DSA is available as a useful aid.

Ideally only nonionic (X-ray) CM should ever be used; on the basis of the study results so far available but as soon as they are on the market, nonionic dimers might be considered in problem cases. Although any CM can lead to reactions, they are both qualitatively less pronounced and quantitatively fewer with the nonionic ICM.

Although reactions remain unpredictable and the known tests have their own complication rate and may be misleading, generous use should be made of prophylactic measures (see Sects. 5.5, 5.6). Since, according to Lalli, the patient's anxiety quite often makes him susceptible to reactions, particular importance also attaches to the physician's explanatory consultation with the patient.

It goes without saying that an exact record must be kept of the examination and of any severe reactions which might occur.

References

1. Lalli AF (1974) Urographic contrast media reactions and anxiety. Radiology 152:267–271

9.4 Phlebography

B. Hagen

The Status of Phlebography

The differential diagnosis of venous disorders is still not achievable without phlebography. Despite the development of sophisticated and noninvasive competing procedures such as scintiscanning with ^{125}I-fibrinogen, isotope phlebography, impedance plethysmography, phlebodynamometry and Doppler sonography, most investigators agree that phlebography is superior to all other procedures in its morphological precision and specificity [2, 3, 6].

Indications

1. Superficial venous system:
   –Complete or incomplete trunk varicosities
   –Suitability of the great saphenous vein for reconstructive surgery
   –Insufficiency of the perforating veins
2. Deep venous system:
   –Acute thrombosis
   –Postphlebitic syndrome
   –Compression syndrome
   –Vascular malformations
   –Monitoring of fibrinolytic therapy
   –Questions requiring a statement of expert opinion

Contraindications

1. Absolute: none
2. Relative
   –Severe anaphylactoid reactions during a previous CM injection
   –Phlegmasia cerulea dolens

Preconditions (see Sect. 9.3)

Methods

Lower extremities and pelvis
1. Ascending leg–pelvis phlebography, phleboscopy (after May and Nissl)
2. Ascending phlebography by Compression (after Hach) [8]
3. Retrograde compression phlebography (following Gullmo) [8]
4. Varicography (after May)
5. DSA of the pelvic veins

Phleboscopy by the method of May and compression phlebography by the method of Hach are standard procedures today for the visualization of the veins of the lower extremity. It is to be emphasized that the visualization of the pelvic veins should always be an integral component of every phlebography of the lower extremity. Since these two methods define not only the morphology of the veins, but also provide functional information (e. g. direction of CM flow in the perforating veins), conventional film techniques (cassette film or a photospot [e. g. 100 mm] camera) should be employed. The pelvic veins, the inferior vena cava and the veins of the upper extremity and shoulder girdle (including the mediastinal veins) can, however, also be visualized using the DSA technique. One can forego puncturing the femoral vein in favour of the less invasive, pedal approach DSA of the pelvic veins and the vena cava. Even though the sharpness of detail is limited in this technique and susceptibility to artefacts is increased, in most cases it is nevertheless sufficient for making a satisfactory diagnosis (Fig. 9.4.1). Only in selective examinations (e. g. of the internal iliac vein, azygos vein, or of the renal or suprarenal vein) and in therapeutic interventions (varicocele treatment, cava filter, stent) are catheterizations via pelvic veins required.

Procedure

Via one of the numerous veins on the dorsum of the foot, a nonionic, low-osmolar CM, the quantity of which is adjusted to the indication and body weight (usually 0.7 ml/kg per extremity), is injected through a butterfly cannula (21 gauge). Standard phlebography under fluoroscopic control comprises three films of the lower leg in external and internal rotation and of the knee-joint region in external rotation for assessing the opening region of the short saphenous vein, two further films of the upper leg

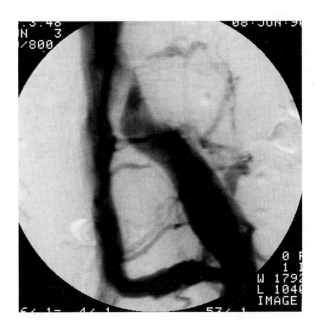

Fig. 9.4.1. Patient (42 years old) with varicosities (left leg). DSA of pelvic veins by pedal injection of 30 ml nonionic CM (300 mg I/ml). Diagnosis: pelvic vein spur

and a film of the pelvis. Valsalva's manoeuvre is used to visualize possible valvular incompetence of the long and short saphenous veins. A tourniquet can be applied briefly above the knee to divert the CM effectively from the superficial into the deep venous system and to assess the perforating veins. After the examination, heparin (2500 IU/extremity) in NaCl infusion solution is administered while the CM is expressed from the varicosities by careful massage of the calf muscles. These physical measures are accompanied by the active dorsal and plantar flexion of the foot. An elastic bandage is then placed around the knee joint and the patient is asked to do walking exercises.

If findings in the pelvic region are unclear a further injection should follow at the same session for DSA of the pelvic veins, where such a system is available. The supine patient is injected with a CM dose of 30 ml (300 mg I/ml), which is followed by an equal volume of physiological saline solution, at a rate of ca. 3–5 ml/s. In order to eliminate intestinal movement artefacts, the injection is preceeded by the administration of 20 mg Buscopan.

Complications

Examination-Induced Complications

With anticoagulation or fibrinolysis, local haematoma can develop at the puncture site, especially if intravascular pressure is increased by the use of a tourniquet. Pain, primarily from multiple puncture attempts or under conditions of orthostasis, can lead to vasovagal disturbances and fainting, especially in younger patients. Given recent thrombosis, one should forego the Valsalva manoeuvre and the forced compression of the calf veins. It seams from case reports that thrombus mobilization and subsequent pulmonary embolism can be caused by the examination.

In phlebography performed with a catheter, complications known from arterial examinations can arise, including dissections of the vein wall, perforation, thrombus formation, arteriovenous fistula formation in multiple puncture attempts, and local haematoma (especially in anticoagulated patients).

Contrast Media-Induced Injuries

Accidental injections into the venous wall can result in painful dissections. These are to be distinguished from paravasation and extravasation. The use of highly concentrated, hyperosmolar, ionic CM can turn such local complications into severe inflammation and tissue necrosis.

With intravascular CM complications we distinguish between those of a general nature (see corresponding chapter) and those of a specifically local nature. The latter can be acute or delayed in onset. Accordingly, we distinguish between pain during injection, postphlebographic thrombophlebitis of the punctured vein and deep vein thrombosis. These side effects involve variably severe forms of injury to the sensitive venous endothelium.

A harmless and reversible superficial thrombophlebitis of the punctured vein is observed in ca. 20% of the cases following administration of ionic CM [7].

Lea Thomas and McDonald report a 0.5% incidence of clinically relevant postphlebographic thrombosis in a series of 3600 patients [5], but a much higher incidence of initial thrombi or signs of thrombus can be found with scintiscanning with ^{125}I-fibrinogen. Albrechtson and Olsson found fibrinogen accumulation in up to 60% of cases in which ionic, hyperosmolar CM were used [1]. In our own investigations using the same measurement technique but modified examination techniques, we found – in 130 patients (260 exams with a randomized and double-blind test design) – such signs of thrombosis in between 15% and 55% of the cases of ionic CM (depending on the CM concentration) but only in an insignificantly low number of nonionic CM cases [4].

As in the arterial system, CM-induced pain in the veins signals that the endothelial tolerance threshold has been exceeded. The effect is caused primarily by CM hyperosmolality and secondarily by CM chemotoxicity. Vascular pain can be reduced through a reduction in concentration, especially of ionic CM. In ionic, monomeric substances, however, a reduction to ca. 150 mg I/ml is necessary to reduce osmolality to a value that is largely free of pain during injection. Nonionic, monomeric or dimeric CM in a concentration up to 250 mg I/ml are tolerated completely without pain [4].

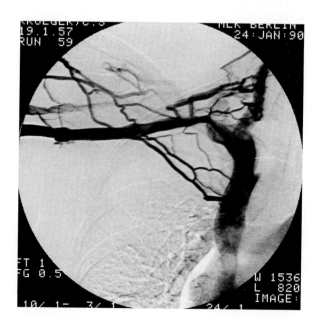

Fig. 9.4.2. Condition of a 33-year-old patient after fibrinolysis of a Paget-v. Schroetter syndrome, progress check. Injection of 15 ml nonionic CM (300 ml I/ml). Diagnosis: restenosis of the subclavian vein at entry to superior vena cava, with collateralization

Conclusion

Phlebography of the lower extremities should be performed as ascending leg-pelvic phlebography by the technique described by May as modified by Hach.

If specifically indicated, the phlebography of the pelvis, the inferior vena cava, and the upper extremity including the shoulder girdle and mediastinum should be carried out using DSA (Fig. 9.4.2). To reduce, objective and subjective unpleasant local side effects, only nonionic CM in a reduced concentration of ca. 250 mg I/ml should be used in phlebography, since the tolerance of the venous endothelium is least challenged in this way. The fact that phlebography is less invasive, employs modern CM that are well tolerated, and displays high diagnostic quality have enabled it to sustain its central role in angiographic diagnosis despite the development of competing procedures.

References

1. Albrechtsson U, Olsson CG (1979) Thrombosis after phlebography: a comparison of two contrast media. Cardiovasc Radiol 2:9–18
2. Bettmann MA, Paulin S (1977) Leg phlebography: the incidence, nature and modification of undesirable side effects. Radiology 122:101–104
3. Hach W (1985) Phlebographie der Bein- und Beckenvenen, 3rd edn. Schnetztor, Konstanz
4. Hagen B (1985) Die Objektivierung der Endothelverträglichkeit nicht-ionischer Kontrastmittel mit dem Radio-Iod-Fibrinogentest bei der Phlebographie. In: Zeitler E (ed) Klinische Pharmakologie der Kontrastmittel. Schnetztor, Konstanz, pp 94–105
5. Lea Thomas M, Mc Donald LM (1978) Complications of ascending phlebography of the leg. BMJ 2:317–318
6. May R, Nißl R (1973) Die Phlebographie der unteren Extremitäten, 2nd edn. Thieme, Stuttgart
7. May R (1977) Thrombophlebitis nach Phlebographie. Vasa 6:169
8. Weber J, May R (1990) Funktionelle Phlebologie. Thieme Verlag

9.5 Direct Lymphography and Indirect Lymphangiography

H. Weissleder

Why?

The noninvasive imaging examination procedures of US, CT, MRT and quantitative radionuclide imaging of the lymph vessels have largely replaced lymphography as routine diagnostic methods [12]. However, morphological changes in epifascial lymph vessels and lymph nodes situated along them may still only be delineated by lymphographic methods.

The sharpness of detail in these procedures is still clearly superior to that of other examination techniques [13].

For the assessment of centrally located lymphatics, lymph nodes and the thoracic duct, oily CM have to be used (direct lymphography) [3, 8]. Because of its known complications, however, the use of this technique is only advisable if there is a clear indication. In general, lymphography should not be performed if any worsening of the disease from the side effects of the examination may be anticipated.

For contrast visualization of the peripheral lymphatics in the extremities, the trunk, and the face and neck region, nonionic, dimeric, water-soluble, iodinated CM that are tolerated well are indicated (indirect lymphangiography) [5–7, 14, 15, 17]. Operative exposure and direct puncture of lymph vessels is not required for this examination.

When?

As a rule, lymphographic examinations represent the last stage of the diagnostic process. In malignant diseases of the lymphatic system, assessment is usually possible by means of US, CT and/or MRI. Direct lymphography with oily CM is only indicated if these other imaging procedures do not provide definitive information.

In primary lymphostatic oedema of the extremities, the use of oily CM is, other than for a handful of exceptions, obsolete and to be viewed as malpractice. Direct lymphography is only acceptable today in the case of a few very specific questions whose answers have therapeutic implications (in a preoperative examination, for example).

For assessing morphological changes in peripheral lymphatics, indirect lymphangiography with water-soluble CM is to be considered the method of choice [14, 15, 18]. In contrast to direct lymphography, it usually also provides an assessment of all primary lymph vessels and precollectors in the body surface region. The technique does not require exposure of peripheral lymphatics and thus is technically much easier to perform; examinations take less time and require less instrumentation.

At the present time, the use of indirect lymphangiography is concentrated on localized and generalized soft tissue swellings of the extremities and the trunk associated with primary or secondary lymphoedema or their combined forms such as lipolymphoedema or phlebolymphoedema [5, 6, 16].

Premises

1. In general, an initial examination providing a basic clinical diagnosis is mandatory before all lymphangiographic examinations. In addition, one should have the results of preceding US, X-ray diagnostic, radio-isotope, and MRI examinations.
2. As in other examinations involving iodinated X-ray CM, their use is relatively contraindicated in latent or manifest hyperthyroidism or in known CM allergies. Contraindications to X-ray exposure should also be considered.

Methods

Direct Lymphography

1. The upper extremities: for visualizing the epifascial lymph collectors and axillary lymph nodes, the oily CM is infused into an exposed lymph vessel on the back of the hand. CM infusions on the palmar aspect of the distal forearm are also possible.
2. The lower extremities, pelvic and lumbar lymph nodes, throracic duct: for visualizing the ventromedial, epifascial, lymph vessel bundle and the inguino-pelvic and lumbar nodes the CM is infused into a lymph vessel of the back of the foot. By means of a retromalleolar infusion, the collectors of the epifascial, dorsolateral bundle can be demonstrated. To assess subfascial lymph vessels, the CM has to be injected intramuscularly (into the calf muscles).

The technique of CM administration has basically remained unchanged since the introduction of direct lymphography [9–11]. After labelling of superficial lymph vessels by means of a subcutaneous injection of dye (patent blue or violet – with attention to side effects), the desired lymphatic is isolated under local anaesthesia. Then, the vessel is punctured with a special cannula. An automatic infusion pump is required for CM administration with an injection rate of 5–10 ml/h. In diseases not accompanied by considerable lymph node enlargement, an infusion of 5 ml per lower extremity may be sufficient. As a rule, undesirable side effects result from larger volumes. In the region of the upper extremities, 2–3 ml CM usually suffices to fill the lymphatics and regional lymph nodes.

During infusion of oily CM, pain along the course of the epifascial lymphatics may occur if there is an imbalance between vessel capacity and infusion rate. This pain results from rupture of the vascular wall. In such cases, the rate of infusion should be reduced or the infusion interrupted for a short time. If allergic reactions occur, it is necessary to stop the CM infusion and initiate appropriate treatment without delay.

After completing the CM infusion, anteroposterior (AP) X-ray films are made of the extremities and of the trunk at two levels (the lymphangiogram comprises the filling phase). In order to visualize the lymph nodes free of any superimposition, the same series of films is repeated ca. 24 h later (the lymphadenogram comprises the storage phase).

Indirect Lymphangiography

A subepidermal infusion of appropriate, water-soluble CM permits the visualization of peripheral lymphatics, and incompetence of the lymphatic valves. It also permits an assessment of primary lymph vessels [7]. The CM is generally infused into toes, fingers or into the backs of the feet or hands.

Other injection sites are possible, depending on the clinical question posed. In localized oedema, for example, the CM can also be infused into the face and neck region or in the trunk.

The diagnostic value of visualization of the peripheral lymphatics is largely dependent upon injection technique. This, in turn, is firmly based upon accurate subepidermal positioning of the cannula tip. Following puncture, the cannula tip should remain just visible through the skin. During infusion, an epidermal wheal is produced with a dark centre and a lighter border. This indicates accurate cannula location.

The infusion rate is on the average, 0.15 ml/min. Slower infusions lead to decreased contrast density in the lymph vessels. A total amount of 2–4 ml CM per puncture site is sufficient.

Peripheral lymphatics and, under certain conditions, dilated primary lymph vessels also can usually be demonstrated a few minutes after infusion begins. The first X-ray film is made 3–5 min after the start of infusion in order to register local changes in the area of the puncture site. Later, these changes may be overshadowed by the CM collection and thus escape detection. In addition, films should be taken at intervals of ca. 5 min until the desired area is visualized. In contrast to the case with direct lymphography, however, lymphatics can only be assessed here over a length of approximately 40 cm. This is the result of the relatively rapid diffusion of CM through the vessel wall. Visualization of the lymph nodes is not possible with indirect lymphangiography.

Complications I: Those Induced by the Method

Direct Lymphography

Wound infections, delayed healing of wounds, lymphangitis, erysipelas, and cutaneous necrosis are side effects that have to be reckoned with in direct lymphography [1]. Inaccurate positioning of the cannula can lead to extravasation and unwanted CM intravasation in neighbouring veins. The frequency of allergic reactions to the dye used, patent blue/violet, is put at 0.1%–1.5%. Allergic reactions can also be triggered by skin desinfectants [1].

Indirect Lymphangiography

No complications of indirect lymphangiography are presently known. A slight burning sensation during infusion in the area of the puncture on one or both sides was commented (on by ca. 10% of the 150 patients of our own series. It was never necessary to interrupt the examination. If pain becomes intolerable, however, the infusion rate should be reduced. The burning sensation is not induced by the CM, but is a result of local tissue irritation by the interstitial infusion. In isolated cases, small cutaneous ulcers have been observed in the area of puncture. They healed in a few days without treatment and without sequelae.

Complications II: Those Induced by the Contrast Medium

Direct Lymphography

Allergic reactions to the oily, iodinated CM are to be expected in 1:800 examinations on the basis of accumulated data. CM-induced foreign-body reactions with subsequent fibrosis of the lymph nodes [4] and paravascular foreign-body reactions in cases of extravasation can lead to a reduction of the transport capacity of the lymphatic system. In lymphostatic oedemas of the extremities, this usually results in a worsening of the disease. Passage of the oily CM into the venous system results in microemboli in the lung [1, 2]. There is a direct relationship between the frequency of pulmonary complications (Table 9.5.1) and the CM dose administered. Volumes of less than 3.5 ml per lower extremity are usually well tolerated. Lung diseases accompanied by marked limitation of function are to be viewed as contraindications to direct lymphography. Cerebral, renal and cardiac complications (1:2700–5000) are possible, though rare. CM passage into the liver usually has no sequelae. According to the literature, temporary temperature rises (dose dependent) have to be reckoned with in 10%–20% of examinations [1]. The frequency of nausea and vomiting is put at 4%.

Table 9.5.1. Pulmonary complications and deaths after direct lymphography with oily CM. Results from two composite statistical studies based on 32 000 and 40 500 examinations, respectively

Complications or deaths	Study results	
	Keinert [1]	Köhler and Viamonte [2]
Pulmonary embolism	1: 400	1: 1400
Lipiodol pneumonia	1:2500	1: 1900
Pulmonary oedema	1:3200	1:10 000
Death	1:1800	1:13 500

Indirect Lymphangiography

Allergic reactions triggered by nonionic CM are possible, though rare (see Sects. 4.1, 4.2). Nothing is presently known about other CM-induced complications.

Conclusions

Since the use of oily CM can lead to severe complications, direct lymphography should only be performed if valuable diagnostic information will be gained from it and procedures involving lower risk have not produced an unequivocal diagnosis. The routine use of oily CM is no longer justified today. Direct lymphography is contraindicated if a worsening of the disease can be expected from the side effects associated with the examination. This can generally be assumed to be the case in primary lymphoedema. For the visualization of lymphatics in peripheral regions (indirect lymphangiography), nonionic, dimeric, water-soluble, X-ray CM that are well-tolerated should be exclusively used.

References

1. Keinert K, Köhler K, Platzbecker H (1983) Komplikationen und Kontraindikationen. In: Lüning M, Wiljasalo M, Weissleder H (eds) Lymphographie bei malignen Tumoren. Thieme, Stuttgart
2. Koehler PR, Viamonte Jr M (1980) „Complications". In: Viamonte M Jr, Rüffimann M (eds) Atlas of lymphography. Thieme, Stuttgart
3. Lüning M, Wiljasalo M, Weissleder H (1983) Lymphographie bei malignen Tumoren. Thieme, Stuttgart
4. Oehlert W, Weissleder H, Gollasch D (1966) Lymphogramm und histologisches Bild bei normalen und pathologisch veränderten Lymphknoten. RÖFO 104:751–758
5. Partsch H, Stöberl C, Urbanek A, Wenzel-Hora B (1988) Die indirekte Lymphographie zur Differentialdiagnose des dicken Beines. Phlebol Prokt 17:3–10
6. Partsch H, Stöber C, Wruhs M, Wenzel-Hora B (1989) Indirect lymphography with iotrolan. Recent developments in nonionic contrast media. In: Taenzer, Wende (eds) Thieme, Stuttgart 178–181
7. Stöberl C, Partsch H (1988) Indirekte Lymphographie. Ödem 105–107
8. Viamonte M Jr, Rüttimann A (1980) Atlas of lymphography. Thieme, Stuttgart
9. Viamonte M Jr, Rüttimann A (1980) Technique. In: Viamonte M Jr, Rüttimann A (eds) Atlas of Lymphography. Thieme, Stuttgart
10. Weissleder H (1965) Die Lymphographie. Ergeb Inn Med Kinderheilk 23:297–334
11. Weissleder H (1981) Lymphographie. In: Frommhold W(ed). Erkrankungen des Lymphsystems. Thieme, Stuttgart
12. Weissleder H (1986) Stellenwert der direkten Lymphographie. Ödem 68–76
13. Weissleder H (1988) Aktueller Stand bildgebender Verfahren in der Lymphödemdiagnostik. Ödem 42–48
14. Weissleder H (1990) Zwei schonende Methoden der Lymphgefäßdiagnostik. Herz Gefasse 10:8–16
15. Weissleder H, Weissleder R (1989) Interstitial lymphography: initial clinical experience using a dimeric non-ionic contrast agent. Radiology 170:371–374
16. Weissleder H, Weissleder R (1989) Vergleichende indirekte Lymphangiographie und Lymphszintigraphie bei Lymphödemen der Extremitäten. Lymphologica 71–77
17. Wenzel-Hora B, Partsch H, Berens von Rautenfeld D (1985) Simultane indirekte Lymphographie. In: Holzmann H, Altmeyer P, Hör G, Hahn K (eds) Dermatologie und Nuklearmedizin. Springer, Berlin Heidelberg New York
18. Wenzel-Hora B, Partsch H, Urbanek A (1985) Indirect lymphography with lotasul. The initial lymphatics. 1:117–122

9.6 Angiography and Thoracic Aortography

P. Romaniuk

Why?

In the past 10 years, structural and functional studies of the heart, coronary arteries, and blood vessels have reached a new level of precision.

Invasive examinations of the heart and the major blood vessels make it possible – by means of catheterization, pressure readings, intravascular administration of indicators, and angiocardiography – to clarify complicated anatomy and to determine functional parameters with great precision. Moreover, invasive methods are indispensable exploratory and monitoring tools *before, during* and *after* therapeutic procedures.

Interventional therapy (such as valvuloplasty or percutaneous transluminal angioplasty; PTCA) cannot be performed without being preceded or accompanied by diagnostic angiocardiography or angiography.

When?

Catheterization of the heart and angiocardiography of the cardiac chambers and central vessels is indicated for the following problems:
- Diseases of the pericardium
- Diseases of the myocardium
- Diseases of the cardiac valves
- Cardiac arrhythmia
- Congenital cardiac defects
  - Isolated defects (e. g. ventricular septal defects, VSD)
  - Combined defects (e. g. VSD and patent ductus arteriosus)
  - Complex defects (e. g. tetralogy of Fallot)
- Degenerative diseases of the aorta and the brachiocephalic vessels
- Inflammatory diseases of the aorta and the brachiocephalic vessels
- Traumatic lesions of the aorta and the brachiocephalic vessels
- Congenital aortic defects

Before invasive procedures are used, a range of clinical information and data should be gathered, the state of the patient permitting:
- A short case history
- Physical examination: state, state of vessels (findings from palpation, laboratory tests, Doppler US)
- Resting electrocardiogram
- Electrocardiographic stress test (if necessary, with ergo-oximetry)
- Recorded ECG (Holter monitoring)

- Plain chest X-ray
- Echocardiogram
- Myocardial scintiscan
- Scintiscans of other organs (if necessary)
- CT of the heart (if necessary)
- MRI of the heart (if necessary).

Moreover, a planned catheter procedure requires the following information to permit an estimation of risk and to prepare for complications:
- Blood group
- Coagulation status
- Erythrocyte sedimentation rate
- Findings indicative of organ disease (e. g. hepatic enzymes, creatinine level, metabolic parameters, potassium level and similar readings)
- Bacteriological – serological findings
- Haematological – oncological information (platelet count, leucocyte count, information on tumours and metastases).

Further indispensable information includes
- Current drug therapy (calcium antagonists, beta blockers, cardiac agents, diuretic agents, antiarrhythmic agents)
- The type and function of cardiac pacemakers
- The risk-factor profile (e. g. blood cholesterol values, uric acid level, blood-glucose level).

In a modern cardiological unit, the following is not possible without catheterization:
- Planning of a venous bypass
- Planning an internal mammary coronary graft
- Planning of cardiac valve operations
- Planning of palliative or reconstructive interventions in the case of complex, congenital defects
- Planning of interventional procedures on the coronary arteries, cardiac valves and pericardium.

The following angiocardiographic data are basic to the planning of therapy:
- State of the coronary arteries
- Detection of coronary artery lesions accompanying mitral or aortic valve defects
- Special morphological information on the right and left heart chambers (deformations of chamber shape, e. g. in restrictive cardiomyopathies and similar conditions)
- Heart chamber volumes in end diastole and end systole (comparison with age-related normal values)
- Global and regional ejection fractions of the chambers
- Median (or maximum) fibre contraction rates

- Wall thickness and heart mass
- Cardiac output, cardiac index, cardiac work and cardiac performance
- Determination of the severity of aortic valve stenoses, aortic valve insufficiencies, mitral valve stenoses, mitral insufficiencies; gradation of combined aortic mitral defects; gradation of tricuspid defects
- Depiction of the wall structure of epicardium and pericardium in pericardiac diseases (CM administration following pericardiac puncture or pericardiac drainage)
- Effectivity assessment after pulmonary, mitral, or aortic valvuloplasty.

Other functional parameters can be defined in conjunction with cardiac
catheterization and angiocardiography:
- Pressure values (contractility indices)
- Oxygen saturation values in all heart cavities
- Resistance in the systemic and pulmonary circulations
- Heart minute output (HMO), cardiac index, stroke volume and stroke
  work
- Median (maximum) wall tension in end diastole and end systole
- Systematic and pulmonary resistance.

The following approach facilitates the analysis of complex heart defects by
means of a procedure of segmental analysis.

The following individual questions have to be answered in the angiocardio-
graphic analysis of complex cardiac defects:
- Position of the heart in the thorax (levocardia or dextrocardia? levover-
  sion or dextroversion?)
- Topology of the atria
- Type of venoatrial connection
- Morphology of the atria
- Topology of the chambers
- Type of atrioventricular connection
- Valvular morphology in concordant or discordant atrioventricular connec-
  tion
- Morphology of the chambers
- Morphology of the outflow tract
- Topology of the major vessels
- Type of ventriculoarterial (ventriculovenous) connection
- Morphology of the ascending aorta and the coronary arteries
- Morphology of the aortic arch and the descending aorta
- Morphology of the pericardium
- Structures of shunt defects (morphology of the atrial septum, morphology
  of the ventricular septum, morphology of the truncus region, morphology
  of the ductal region)
- Structure of atypical shunt defects

– Collateral circulations (arteriovenous shunts, systemic – pulmonary shunts)
– Structure of surgically produced bypasses

In answering these questions, a series of special, structural lesions have to be evaluated in the angiocardiogram for the individual heart defects. They are summarized as follows for each defect:

Pulmonary Valve Stenosis

– Precise determination of the anatomical relationships of subvalvular–muscular, valvular, and supravalvular constriction of the chambers and of the pulmonary trunk
– Angiographic clarification of the pulmonary circulation (single or multiple pulmonary stenoses?)
– Classification of the type of pulmonary stenosis (e. g. characterization of valvular dysplasias)
– Functional evaluation of right ventricular strain

Aortic Valve Stenosis

– Precise morphological clarification of the valvular lesion and the left-ventricular outflow channel (e. g. delineation of accompanying membranous, semilunar, subvalvular structures; delineation of dystopias of the anterior mitral valvular cusp, detection of accessory valvular tissue, clarification of the geometry of the left-ventricular outflow tract)

Ventricular Septal Defect

– Precise localization of VSD (inflow tract defect, perimembranous, high or low muscular localization; infracristal, supracristal defect, multiple defects)
– Angiocardiographic estimation of the size of the defect and of the left-right shunt
– Estimated haemodynamic parameters (pressure behaviour in the cardiac cavities, wall motion, local contractility, HMV and cardiac index, resistance values)

Atrial Septal Defect

– Clarification of questionable, accompanying transposition of pulmonary veins
– Oximetric or angiocardiographic clarification of left transposition of the inferior vena cava (accompanying larger atrial septal defects, ASD)

Atrial Septal Defect Ventricular Septal Defect

– Rarely-occurring defect combinations that require precise angiocardiographic estimation of the size of ASD and VSD components
– Visual, angiocardiographic estimation of shunt volumes

Ventricular Septal Defect and Ductus Arteriosus

– Morphological clarification of the size and localization of the VSD and of the size and shape of the ductal canal

Patent Ductus Arteriosus

– Angiocardiographic clarification of ductal anatomy, the structure of the thoracic aorta, and the relationship to the brachiocephalic vessels

Valvular Pulmonary Stenosis, Atrial Septal Defect, and Persistent Left Superior Vena Cava

– Angiocardiographic and haemodynamic diagnosis as above.
– Since in operations using heart – lung machines, persistent left superior vena cava trigger constant bleeding with their communicating vessels and obscure the heart site, CM should be injected into the left subclavian vein, in order to define the deformation.

Valvular Aortic Stenosis and Patent Ductus Arteriosus

– Angiocardiographic diagnosis as given above

Atrioventricular Septal Defect (Types A–C, Special Form)

– Exact differentiation – by means of angiocardiography – of the ASD and VSD components, the defect of the anterior atrioventricular (AV) cusp system (free-floating, common anterior cusp; fixated, common anterior cusp; split, septally fixated, anterior cusp system; lesions of the posterior cusp system), wall motion, and components of insufficiency
– In addition, clarification of the morphology of the pulmonary arteries and veins required

Persistent Truncus Arteriosus (Types I–III)

– Clarification of the aortic origins of pulmonary vessels crucial for operative correction

– Further foci of CM examination: ventriculography for clarifying accompanying defects (e. g. VSD) and for determining chamber volume and cardiac function

Ebstein's Anomaly

– Clarification of complex deformed anatomy of the tricuspid valve (minor caudal dislocation of valve in its position vis-a-vis annulus fibrosus or major dislocation in position of membranously deformed AV valve) for purposes of quantification
– Comprehensive hemodynamic studies are also to be included.

Cor Triatriatum

– Rare defect, difficult to recognize. The stenotic membrane formation in the left atrium necessitates angiocardiography depicting the parts of the left atrium as well as the pulmonary vascular system.

Complete Transposition of Great Vessels

– In the case of the complete (dextro; d-)transposition of great vessels, i. e. the complete reversal of the exits of great vessels from the cardiac chambers with accompanying ASD, VSD, patent ductus arteriosus, aortic isthmus stenosis and, more rarely, with complete AV septal defects (in different variations), it is imperative that
    – Angiocardiography of both chambers of the heart, including pressure analysis and angiocardiography of the aorta and pulmonary arteries be performed for verification of the defect
– Without angiocardiography, no acute, life-sustaining interventions (balloon atrial septostomy, septectomy, switch operations) are possible.

Corrected Transposition of Great Vessels

– In the corrected (levo; I-)transposition of great vessels, which is anatomically compensated for by an inversion of chamber position, angiocardiography for clarification of additional, accompanying defects (valvular and subvalvular pulmonary stenosis, VSD) is indicated.

Double Outlet Syndrome

The syndromes in which both major vessels (aorta and pulmonary trunk) originate from *one* chamber can be divided into two groups:

– Double outlet right ventricle syndrome
– Double outlet left ventricle syndrome.

The angiocardiographic analysis of the *double outlet right ventricle syndrome* focuses on the following special anatomical features:
– Is there a d-transposition or a d-malposition of the major vessels?
– Is the aorta (in a d-malposition) completely or incompletely transposed?
– Is the pulmonary trunk (in an L-malposition) completely or incompletely transposed?
– Is there an additional pulmonary valve stenosis (combined valvular – subvalvular)?
– Is there a VSD?
– How is the VSD positioned?
– Is there complicated form of the double outlet right ventricle syndrome (e. g. with an intact ventricular septum and obstruction of the ventricular outflow tract, with VSD and subaortal obstruction, in combination with transposition of pulmonary veins)

The angicardiography clarification of a *double outlet left ventricle syndrome* largely follows the guidelines given above:
– Clarification of the malposition of the major vessels
– Clarification of the transposition of the major vessels
– Clarification of VSD anatomy
– Clarification of additional, complex deformations.

Fallot Deformation Complex

– Angiocardiography in the case of Fallot's tetralogy serves to:
  – Determine chamber volume (comparison of volume with age-related ideal values)
  – Determine cardiac function (contractility, ejection fraction values, wall motion of both chambers)
  – Determine the morphology of the pulmonary valve and the right ventricular outflow tract
  – Determine the relationship of the diameters of the pulmonary trunk and aorta
  – Clarify the pulmonary vessel periphery

Aortic Deformations

All forms of:
– *Aortic deformations* (persistent truncus arteriosus communis, *pseudotruncus ateriosus*)
– Aortopulmonary *septal defects*

– Incomplete or complete *double aortic arches*
– *Aortic isthmus stenosis* (pre- and postductal forms)
– *Aortic arch hypoplasia* (including aortic isthmus atresia) and
– *Anomalies* of the brachiocephalic vessels, continue to be diagnosed invasively and by means of angiocardiography (due to imaging problems in echocardiography and to the difficulties of interpretation of morphological details).

Pulmonary Atresia

Atresia of the pulmonary trunk is classified in types A–D according to the degree of defect (atresia of the pulmonary valve; atresia of the pulmonary valve and pulmonary trunk with completely intact, central pulmonary vessels; atresia of the pulmonary valve, pulmonary trunk and central pulmonary trunks; and atresia of the pulmonary valve, pulmonary trunk, pulmonary trunks, and the central regions of the segmental arteries).
– Angiocardiographic diagnosis focuses on the definitive clarification of the type of pulmonary atresia of the morphology of the left and right chambers and on the pulmonary vessel periphery.

Tricuspidal Atresia

Angiocardiographic diagnosis concentrates on:
– Clarification of the anatomical structures of the right side of the heart (size of the right atrium, size of the ASD chamber volume, detection of subvalvular stenosis)
– Clarification of the pulmonary vascular system (e. g. additional, peripheral pulmonary stenosis)
– Clarification of the structures and dynamics of the left heart chamber (working chamber).

Angiocardiographically, tricuspidal atresias can be subdivided into the following types:

Type I: Tricuspidal atresia with normal aortas and pulmonary arteries (Ia with pulmonary valve stenosis, Ib with pulmonary valve hypoplasia, Ic with normal pulmonary valve and VSD)

Type II: Tricuspid atresia with d-transposition of the major vessels (IIa with pulmonary valve atresia, IIb with valvular – subvalvular pulmonary stenosis and VSD, IIc with normal pulmonary valve and VSD)

Type III: Tricuspidal atresia with A-transposition of the major vessels (IIIa with valvular – subvalvular pulmonary stenosis without VSD, IIIb with subvalvular pulmonary stenosis and VSD, IIIc in combination with more complex defects).

Hypoplastic Left-Heart Syndrome

The term syndrome is generally only allowed in the case of the simultaneous occurrence of lesions on the mitral valve, mitral valve apparatus, papillary musculature, left-ventricular free chamber wall, aortic valve, ascending aorta and aortic isthmus.

In order of frequency, the deformation occurs in the following combinations:
– Mitral-valve hypoplasia and aortic atresia
– Mitral-valve dysplasia and aortic-valve stenosis
– Mitral-valve stenosis and aortic-valve stenosis
– Mitral-valve insufficiency, subvalvular aortic stenosis and valvular aortic stenosis
– Mitral insufficiency, aortic-valve insufficiency, valvular aortic stenosis and aortic-isthmus stenosis, and
– Mitral-valve atresia and aortic-isthmus stenosis.

The CM examination concentrates on the following details:
– Shape of the pulmonary arteries
– Right–left shunt in ductal area
– Shape of the pulmonary veins
– Extent of retrograde circulation via the ductus arteriosus
– Size and form of the left atrium
– Type of mitral-valve lesion
– Lesions of the tendinous cords or papillary musculature
– Lesions of the aortic valve (aortic-valve atresias, subvalvular region, extreme subvalvular hypoplasias)
– Perfusion capacity of the coronary vessels
– Definitive anatomy of the thoracic aorta.

Cardiomyopathies

As stipulated by the WHO, cardiomyopathies are divided into idiopathic and specific forms. Idiopathic cardiomyopathies are divided into hypertrophic forms (including hypertrophic-obstructive states), dilatative forms, and restrictive forms.

Cardiomyopathies that arise following myocarditis or other inflammatory lesions (rheumatism, tuberculosis, collagen diseases) are designated specific forms.

Fibroelastosis and myocardial diseases due to storage diseases (e. g. glycogen storage disease) are special forms of childhood cardiomyopathies that are difficult to classify.
– In all forms of cardiomyopathies, invasive and angiocardiographic diagnosis is indicated to clarify chamber geometry, chamber volume, cardiac function and the state of coronary vessels. Invasive diagnosis is frequently supplemented by a myocardial biopsy.

Cardiac Tumours

By analogy, the principles of invasive diagnosis of congenital and acquired defects (cardiac catheterization, angiocardiography, coronary angiography) also apply for clarifying rare cardiac tumours (atrial myxoma, fibromyoma of the heart chambers, myocardial sarcoma).

Thoracic Aorta and Brachiocephalic Vessels

Catheter diagnosis with angiography of the thoracic aorta and the brachiocephalic vessels is indicated for:
– Anomalies of origin and location
– Suspected occlusive vascular lesions (main symptoms: murmurs, variations in pulse, transitory ischaemic attacks, intermittent blindness, insufficiencies in basilar or vertebral circulations or complete strokes). Arteriosclerosis, thrombosis, embolism, dissections of the aorta, independent dissections of the brachiocephalic vessels, fibromuscular dysplasia, neurovascular compression syndromes, arteritis syndromes and lesions following irradiation are causes of occlusive lesions.
– Aneurysmal lesions
– Aortic ectasia
– Effects of trauma (arteriovenous fistula, false aneurysma, vascular wall lacerations)
– Postoperative effects (restenosis following operation, aneurysms following operation, para-aortic bleeding, lesions of the spinal arteries, aneurysms of the bronchial arteries, restenosis following endarterioectomies)
– Tumours: bronchial carcinoma (infiltrations of the azygos vein or intercostal veins), haemangioma (thoracic wall, throat, face, shoulder region), nasopharyngeal angiofibroma, thyroidal carcinoma, parathyroidal adenoma
– Paraganglioma
– Dislocation, compression, infiltration of vessels by laryngeal tumours, hypopharyngeal tumours or cervical metastases
– Vascular anomalies (variants of origin of brachiocephalic vessels, collateral circulation).

Angiocardiographies Accompanying Cardiac Interventions

Angiographic or angiocardiographic examinations are used as exploratory tools for all the following interventions:
– Balloon atrial septostomy according to Rashkind
– Percutaneous duct closure according to Porstmann or Rashkind
– Percutaneous valvotomy
– Percutaneous angioplasty of the aorta

– Embolization therapy
– Angioplasties of the brachiocephalic vessels
– Angioplasties of intracranial branches
– Embolization (AV fistula, AD deformations, traumatic bleeding, epistaxis, tumours, stent implantations, embolization of parathyroidal andenoma, embolization of angioma of the throat).

Invasive Diagnosis in Hormonally Active Tumours

In addition to venous and arterial angiography (thyroid region, parathyroid region, throat region, mediastinal region), selective blood samples can help make the localization and determination of the size of hormonally active tumours more precise.

Angiography of the Spinal Arteries (see Sect. 9.2)

How?

Cardiac Catheterization and Angiocardiography in Premature Babies, Newborns and Infants

An attempt is made to perform all forms of vascular puncture and catheter introduction for the catheterization of cardiac cavities and angiocardiography under local anaesthetic. Sufficient sedation is a prerequisite for successful puncture and catheterization.

Usually, a *purely venous* approach is sufficient, since all cardiac cavities and major vessels can be reached by means of the open foramen ovale, either through the VSD, the pulmonary trunk (via the patent ductus arteriosus) or by a turning manoeuvre in the left chamber.

A percutaneous puncture should always be attempted (after local anaesthetic and stab incision of the skin). The left groin is a favourable location. If this fails, the femoral vein can still be punctured in the right groin.

The delicate femoral vessel in premature babies, newborns and infants has to be punctured with thin, one–way cannulas (allowing a 0.5-mm guidewire).

The puncture of the femoral vein is made ca. 5 mm below the inguinal ligament, directly medially to the pulsating artery. The femoral vein is exposed by means of a ca. 10-mm-long longitudinal incision, which begins at the level of the inguinal ligament; the great saphenous vein is exposed by means of a transverse incision made about 5 mm distally from the inguinal ligament.

The use of a catheter sheath limits endothelial injury in cases where the catheter is changed several times or catheter manipulation extends over a longer period of time.

In premature babies, newborns and infants, one should avoid catheterization of the femoral *artery* since it can very frequently be accompanied by complications (long–lasting spasm, thrombotic occlusion, peripheral emboli, wall lacerations).

According to procedure used, we distinguish between
– Right cardiac catheterization
– Left cardiac catherization and
– Transseptal cardiac catherization.

In a right cardiac catherization, the inferior and superior vena cava are first catherized and localized. Then the right cardiac chambers (right atrium, right ventricle) are explored or catheterized. Pressure measurements and blood gas tests are included. The pulmonary artery is probed with Cournand-type catheters, ring catheters or balloon catheters.

Before or after the angiocardiography of the heart chambers, calibrations are made in the middle of the heart, e. g. by imaging metal balls, in order to make a morphological measurements possible (determination of volume, ejection fraction, HMO, cardiac index and so on).

With the help of a computer, it is then possible, on the basis of the pressure and blood gas values, to determine shunt volume, cardiac output and cardiac index, as well as vascular resistances. Pigtail catheters that allow for an even distribution of CM in the heart cavities should be used for angiocardiography.

Only nonionic CM are used for the angiography of premature babies, newborns and infants, in order to minimize the risks of decompensation or a haemodynamic or electric destabilization of the heart.

Many authors are sceptical about using digital substraction angiography (DSA) on infants due to:
– Radiation exposure
– Inadequate subtraction due to the rapid movements of the heart.

Nevertheless, DSA technique is of great value for clarifying difficult anatomical structures (such as deformation of the aortic arch and clarification of postoperative aortopulmonary shunts).

As a rule of thumb, the overall CM doses for angiocardiography should not exceed 4 ml/kg, max. 5 ml/kg. Some authors use up to 7 ml/kg, but leave 10–30 min between CM injections and administer additional sedatives during these breaks. The tolerance to CM can be further increased if every angiocardiography is followed by a short infusion of saline in order to accelerate elimination.

The risk of CM side effects are greater, the closer the CM administration is made to the brain (aortic arch!).

If a CM injection into the pulmonary trunk is planned in the case of severe pulmonary hypertension, preliminary oxygen breathing of ca. 5 min. is recommended, in order to avoid possible complications.

Cardiac Catheterization and Angiocardiography in Children

Even though cardiac catheterization and angiocardiography of very severe congenital heart defects in children is not fundamentally different from that used on premature babies, newborns and infants, there are some special features to be observed:

- Since the foramen ovale is closed in children and the path via the ductus arteriosus can no longer be taken, transvenous catherization has to be supplemented by a retrograde, arterial catheterization. If retrograde cha-terization fails (e. g. in severe aortic-valve stenosis), the transseptal proce-dure is used (with needle puncture of the atrial septum).
- Specially formed catheters are used for angiocardiographic imaging (including pressure and blood gas analyses) in a series of special, anatomi-cal questions (origin and course of the coronary arteries, imaging of aortopulmonary collaterals, imaging of surgically placed, aortopulmonary shunts).

Angiocardiography Accompanying Interventional Cardiology Treatments in Children

For the angiocardiographic imaging of cardiac or vascular structures before, during, or after interventional procedures, as little CM as possible should be used, since the interventions themselves (dilatation of the entry vessels, valvotomy procedures in the atrial septum or valves, dilatation of the pul-monary vascular ring, abrupt interruption of shunt circulation, excessive volume and pressure strain in valvuloplasty, ischaemia after embolization) result in considerable cardiocirculatory strain.

Cardiac Catheterization and Angiocardiography in Adults

The following methods are available for introducing the catheter, recording pressure, administering indicators, analyzing blood gas and angiocardiogra-phy of all four cardiac cavities and the major vessels near the heart in adults:

- Right cardiac catheterization
- Left cardiac catherization
- Transseptal cardiac catheterization
- All forms of right cardiac catherization are performed (if no peripheral vessel obstructions exist) percutaneously via the femoral vein. The stan-dard technique for minimizing vascular trauma includes a catheter sheath. In right catherization solely for taking pressure measurements, pigtail catheters can be used; they make a rapid, low-risk study of the right side of the heart possible.
  In more detailed studies (determination of right-ventricular chamber pres-sure, right-ventricular ejection fraction, HMO and cardiac index, as well

as pulmonary pressure, including PC measurements), thermodilution is implemented with special balloon catheters. For the angiocardiography of the right side of the heart (right atrium, right ventricle, pulmonary trunk), only pigtail catheters should be used.

Only in very special morphometric studies (e. g. volume behaviour after heart transplants), for purposes of volume measurement, is angiocardiographic imaging of the right cardiac chamber at two levels used.

– Left cardiac catheterization is also accomplished percutaneously and transfemorally, using a sheath. In complete obstruction of the femoral vessels, a transaxillary approach can be used. If the axillary approach is also unavailable, the left heart chamber can be catheterized transseptally
– Pigtail catheters are usually used for retrograde catherization of the left heart chambers. Coronary catheters (Amplatz left) are alternatives
– An examination of the left atrium is conducted either by turning a pigtail catheter in the left chamber or transseptally
– In cardiomyopathies, the left and right cardiac catheterizations are supplemented by antegrade or retrograde myocardial biopsies
– For imaging the coronary arteries in all main–branch and side–branch vessel areas, three to five injections are required on the left side and at least three on the right side (6–10 ml nonionic CM)
– In very severe, life–threatening conditions (immediately after a myocardial infarction or in the case of unstable angina pectoris with the threat of infarction), invasive diagnosis should be strictly limited to selective coronary arteriography (if necessary, with continuous nitrate infusion and indwelling pacemaker. Nonionic CM are standard.

Angiography of the Aorta and Its Branches

Three procedures are available for imaging the thoracic aorta and its branches:
– Conventional angiography with cine, medium-format, or large-format technique
– Intravenous DSA technique
– Intraarterial DSA technique

Intravenous DSA has not completely satisfied expectations despite many methodological modications (such as CM administration with ring catheters into the right atrium). It is suitable for orienting imaging of the aorta and the brachiocephalic vessels, such as immediately after surgery (e. g. suspected carotid occlusion after endarterioectomy in the area of carotid bifurcation). Venous DSA fails, however, due to its limited imaging quality in the clarification of complex anatomical details, especially in patients with reduced cardiac output and enlarged, central blood volume. In very severely ill patients, due to the relatively large amount of CM it uses, it can lead to symptoms of angina, decompensation of cardiac insufficiency, renal insufficiencies and transitory cerebral ischaemic attacks of the cerebral circulation.

Arterial DSA has proved to be an extremely reliable procedure for defining aortic and vascular lesions. By using modern CM injections through thin, high-flow catheters, optimal imaging can be achieved with a relatively small amount of nonionic CM (ca. 30 ml, containing 300 mg/ml I).

We consider imaging in three stages to be necessary for the preoperative assessment of the aortic region:

Stage 1: Imaging of the aortic arch in 45°–60° left anterior oblique (LAO) views with demonstration of the arch and central region of the brachiocephalic vessels (CM needed: ca. 30 ml, nonionic CM, 300 mg I/ml, flow 15–20 ml/s, injection: ascending aorta)

Stage 2: Imaging of the brachiocephalic vessels at the level of the carotid bifurcation (projection in LAO 45°, CM requirement ca. 30 ml, 300 mg I/ml, injection: ascending aorta)

Stage 3: Imaging of the brachiocephalic vessels and intracranial circulation in anteroposterior projection (injection of ca. 30 ml CM, containing 300 mg I/ml)

This procedure provides imaging of all four cerebral arteries in the neck region, the confluence of the verebral arteries, the basilar artery and the medial and posterior cerebral arteries.

– A lateral projection of the aorta (with 30 ml CM in a flow of 23 ml/s, DSA) is sufficient for clarifying aortic valve insufficiency or aortic valve stenosis.

– Imaging of the thoracic aorta at two levels is recommended for more extensive pathological lesions of the thoracic aorta (aneurysms in the area of the ascending aorta, aortic arch or descending aorta; dissecting aneurysms; local, traumatic laceration of the aortic arch; dissections of the brachiocephalic vessels, Erdheim's cystic medial necrosis, Marfan syndrome). If required, this may be supplemented by oblique-axial projection (LAO and RAO in DSA)

– Special catheter shapes are required for supplementary, selective angiocardiography of the brachiocephalic trunk, of the left and right common carotid artery, the subclavian artery, the left and right vertebral arteries or the individual cerival trunks or mammary arteries. As a rule, 3–5 ml of a nonionic CM per injection are sufficient for DSA

– Specially formed catheters are also used for the study of the external carotid artery, maxillary artery, temporal artery, occipital artery, vertebral artery, thyrocervical trunk, costocervical trunk, superior and inferior thyroid arteries, internal mammary artery and further branches of the shoulder and throat region. As a rule, 2–4 ml of a nonionic CM are sufficient for superselective angiography.

Complications

Technique-Related Complications (See also Sect. 9.3)

- The practitioner with little experience in puncturing femoral vessels in premature babies, newborns and infants should mark vascular axes echographically, in order to avoid mispunctures and consequent haematomas
- Puncture cannulas, guidewires and catheters are never to be used more than once
- Vessels should be exposed only in those regions of the groin where no efforts at puncture have just been made, since escaping blood can make it difficult to locate fine vessels
- In more severely tortuous or slightly stenotic pelvic vessels (venous and arterial system!), one should quickly resort to hydrophilic guidewires (Terumo system)
- Vascular punctures, in which the front *and* back vascular walls are pierced and the needle is then drawn back into the lumen, have become a thing of the past. The penetration of the front vascular suffices for precise punctures and catherization
- Catheter sheath systems should be used as far as possible, in order to facilitate vascular catherization. In elongated or kinked vessels, such sheaths may be impassable after removing the inner catheter. For this reason, a safety wire should always be left in when catheters are changed
- All examinations mentioned in this section require systemic heparinization with 100 IU/kg. A heparinization of 10000 IU is generally required in coronary angiography.
- Heparin should always be intra-arterially administered beneath the aortic arch, but never in the area flowing to the brain (left chamber, ascending aorta), since heparin injures the blood–brain barrier and contributes to side effects in subsequent CM administration
- After a regular examination period (up to 1.5 h), heparinization is neutralized with an iso-equivalent dose of protamine sulphate. In longer exams, the protamine–sulphate dose has to be reduced
- Protamine neutralization should be omitted in arterial catheterization of children and a longer vascular compression period should be accepted
- Heparin infusions for 6–8 h following arterial catheterization are recommended for avoiding complications in children, especially spasm and thromboses
- All commercial catheters have to be rinsed once or twice with saline before they are introduced into the vascular system, since they might contain dust and other foreign substances from production or packaging
- Catheters should not be forced forward (without guidewires) in retrograde aortic or arterial catheterization, since deviations in costal or bronchial arteries can result in injury to the spinal arteries
- Special care must be taken in the catherization and CM administration into the costocervical trunk, thyrocervical trunk, vertebral arteries

and bronchial arteries, due to the danger of injuring to the spinal branches
- Prior to every selective or superselective CM injection, a test CM injection has to be made to determine whether the catheter is stably positioned in the ostium and whether it triggers central or capillary spasm. If spasm occurs, subsequent main injections can lead to dissection, extravasation, lacerations or organ capillary damage
- If a catheter is occluded by wall contact, forced suction can lead to the formation of gas bubbles, which can then result in air emboli on a subsequent injection
- The same suction effect can be triggered by a very rapid withdrawal of guidewires
- Conventional as well as balloon catheters can deviate into the ascending lumbar vein, the renal veins, the hepatic veins and the right atrium in right cardiac catheterization. Forcibly pushing the catheter can produce pain, spasm and vascular performations
- The right atrium has to be carefully explored and catheterized in cardiac catherization, since it can rapidly lead to arrhythmia in the case of endocardial trauma
- Care must be taken in the catherization of stenotic pulmonary valves with subvalvular stenosis, since the right outflow tract tends to spasms and arrhythmia may be triggered when trauma occurs
- Arterial compression bandages should be left on for a max. of 4 h when using no. 9 F catheters, a max. of 3 h with nos. 8 and 9 F catheters, 2 h with nos. 6 and 7 F catheters, and 1 h with children, in order to avoid local thrombosis and peripheral emboli. After the compression bandage is removed, further bed rest (10–24 h, according to catheter diameter) is required. Venous compression bandages should be left on for a max. of 1.5 h
- If the internal jugular vein is punctured (medially to the sternocleidomastoid muscle, laterally to the internal carotid artery), one has to consider that the internal jugular vein can be associated with stenoses, slings and (very rarely) a medial location vis-a-vis the artery, which can impede catheterization or make it impossible.

Contrast Media–Related Complications

- Especially in premature babies, newborns and infants, CM overdoses (with inadequate premedication and insufficient intervals between injections) lead to haemodynamic instability (with decompensation), electrical instability (with tachyarrhythmia), impairment of cerebral blood flow or renal insufficiency
- Dangerous CNS complications are to be expected (restlessness, hyperpexia, cramps), if large amounts of sodium (large volumes of CM) are directly administered into the aorta
- Selective coronary angiography immediately after acute infarction, with the threat of infarction, in unstable angina, at the beginning of an in-

farction and in haemodynamic or electrical instability acceptable only if emergency medical support is available
– In cases of known CM allergies, ca. 200–300 mg of a soluble prednisolone preparation should be given immediately after vessel puncture and catheterization prior to CM administration.

9.7 Angiographic Procedures for the Liver, Spleen, Pancreas and Portal Venous System

W. Rödl

Preparation of the Patient

1. General Preparation

– Written declaration of informed consent of the patient on the day before the examination
– Fasting for at least 4 h prior to examination
– Determination of coagulation status, and of creatinine and urea
– Shaving of the inguinal region or axilla

2. Special Preparations for Abdominal Angiography

– Diet low in fibre and gas-reducing measures on the day before examination. Intestinal hypotonia (1 ampoule Buscopan or Glucagon IV) prior to the CM injection, especially in intra-arterial DSA
– Plain radiograph for exclusion of residual CM in abdomen. Prior information from US, CT and/or MRI.
– In selective transhepatic portal venous catheterization, for the purpose of pancreatic venous sampling, production of a guiding "venous map" of the portal vein by means of indirect mesenteric and splenic portography on the day before examination. Peroral contrast imaging of the gallbladder on the eve of the examination in order to decrease the risk of gallbladder perforation.

Indications and Indication-Specific Angiographic Procedures

In principle, angiography can be performed as standard with a cut-film changer or as intraarterial DSA.

Liver

Coeliac arteriography, selective and superselective hepatic arteriography and superior mesenteric arteriography should be performed to clarify the following questions:

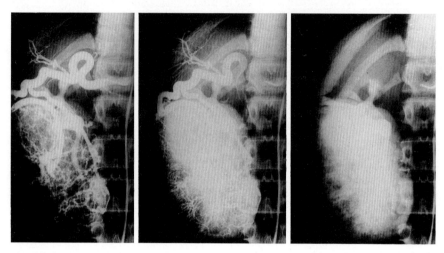

Fig. 9.7.1. Focal nodular hyperplasia of the liver. The richly vascular tumour in the right lobe can be seen in the arterial (a), capillary (b) and parenchymatous phase (c)

- Preoperative vascular anatomy prior to segment resection or transplantation
- Discovery of focal lesions and search for metastases (e. g. vascular metastases in carcinoid (Fig. 9.7.3) or colorectal tumours), discovery of a hepatoma in cirrhosis
- Differential diagnostic classification of vascular tumours such as haemangioma, focal nodular hyperplasia or adenoma, and haemangioendothelioma (Fig. 9.7.2)
- Embolization and/or chemotherapy of liver metastases
- CT portography after selective catheterization of the superior mesenteric artery.

Spleen

Coeliacoarteriography or selective splenic arteriography should be performed in the following situations:
- Preoperative vascular anatomy prior to splenectomy
- Post-traumatic conditions.

Pancreas

Coeliacoarteriography and selective hepatic arteriography or splenic arteriography to answer the following questions:
- Preoperative vascular anatomy, e. g. accessory or replaced hepatic artery prior to a resection of the head of the pancreas
- Differentiation between pancreatitis and carcinoma of the pancreas (vascular encasement)

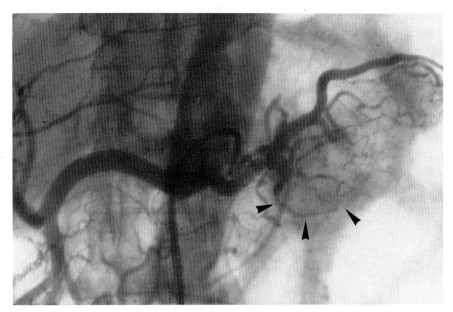

Fig. 9.7.2. Insulinoma of the tail of pancreas. Coeliac angiography demonstrates the round, vascular tumour (arrowheads) which has displaced the vessels in the area of the tail of the pancreases

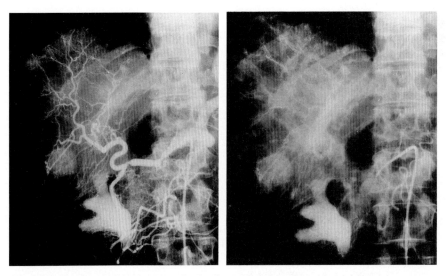

Fig. 9.7.3a, b. Carcinoid metastases in the liver. In the capillary phase (a), but even more impressive in the parenchymatous phase (b), richly vascular carcinoid metastases have been visualized in the liver by selective hepatic arteriography

- In suspected insulinoma: first, superselective angiography of the hepatic artery and/or the gastroduodenal artery on the one hand and of the splenic artery on the other to localize tumours of the head, body or tail of the pancreas (Fig. 9.7.3); secondly, percutaneous, transhepatic portal venous catherization with superselective venous sampling from the veins of the head, body and tail of the pancreas to localize tumours directly
- In suspected gastrinoma: superselective, arterial catherization of the arteries of the head, body and tail of the pancreas. Superselective, intra-arterial secretion (IA-S) stimulation by injection of small doses of secretin (30 units Sekretolin), simultaneous venous sampling, the first time via a transfemoral catheter from the right hepatic vein and then peripherally, from a cubital vein, 30, 60, 120, and 210 s after IA-S stimulation.
An increase in gastrin of over 50% in the 30-s sample from the hepatic vein provides an indirect clue to gastrinoma localization.

Portal Venous System

- In portal hypertension, indirect spleno- and/or mensenteric portography for the differentiation of pre-, intra- and post-hepatic obstruction and for the demonstration of any collateral circulation or hepatofugal flow
- Direct hepatic phlebography in suspected post-hepatic obstruction
- In pancreatic diseases with suspected splenic vein thrombosis and collateral circulation, indirect splenoportography

Contraindications

1. Definite Contraindications

- For puncture, Quick's value under 50%, thrombocyte count under 80,000/cm^3
- For CM injection, creatinine above 2 mg%

2. Relative Contraindications
- General allergic diathesis
- Known CM hypersensitivity
- Known hyperthyroidism
- Patient over 50 years of age with nodular goitre: danger of a compensated, autonomous adenoma with the triggering of a thyreotoxic crisis after CM injection
- Lack of therapeutic implications
- Arterial route of entry (transbrachial, transaxillary) is unsuitable given clinical situation and frequency of complication.

Examination Technique

Puncture and Vascular Approach

1. General
- Local anaesthesia by injection of a 1% local anaesthetic: in transfemoral puncture 10–15 ml, in transaxillary, 10 ml, in transbrachial, 5 ml
- Puncture following skin incision by Seldinger technique. Introduction of a catheter sheath only if multiple catheter change is anticipated and transfemoral approach used

2. In coeliac angiography, selective hepatic angiography, or splenic angiography and in indirect splenic and/or mensenteric angiography, routinely, transfemoral approach: retrograde puncture 3–4 cm below the inguinal ligament.

Only in exceptional cases (stenoses of the iliac arteries or of the adominal aorta, the presence of a bifurcation prothesis or other factors resulting in a higher risk of complications) is a transaxillary approach (right axilla routinely punctured 7 cm laterally of the deepest point of the armpit) or a transbrachial approach (brachial artery in the bend of the elbow above the medial condyle of humerus) utilized.

3. In selective hepatic vein sampling with or without phlebography, routinely a transfemoral approach is used; only in deep vein thrombosis of the leg or pelvis is an ante cubital or transjugular approach used.

4. In selective pancreatic vein sampling (suspected insulinoma) by means of percutaneous, transhepatic, portal venous catheterization, transhepatic approach under fluoroscopic control
- Puncture site is the 9th-11th intercostal space in the midaxillary line, on the right. Direction of puncture: T-12
- Puncture with an in-dwelling catheter needle. Removal of the inner needle. Retraction of the catheter until portal blood drains. Make sure of intraportal catheter position by means of CM injection
- Substitution of a J-wire with a moveable core
- Introduction of a headhunter catheter (5 F) and placement of the catheter tip, first in the splenic hilum, then in the peripheral mesenteric branches
- Stage-by-stage retraction of the catheter accompanied by superselective pancreatic vein sampling at each stage (6–8 ml each time) and by the marking of the sampling position on a venous map previously drawn up (indirect splenomesenteric portography on the previous day)
- Blood samples sent to laboratory for chemical analysis. The topographical correlation of the hormone peak with the sampling location makes insulinoma localization possible (Fig. 9.7.4).

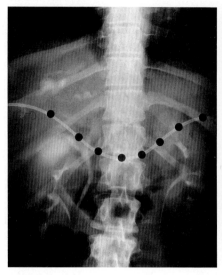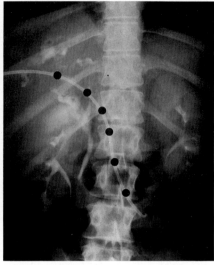

Fig. 9.7.4a, b. Transhepatic portal catheterization in insulinoma. After transhepatic puncture, the catheter is introduced up to the hilus of the spleen and to the root of the mesenteric artery. To determine the hormone level 4–6 ml blood is selectively drawn from the splenic artery (a) and superior mesenteric vein (b) and from the portal confluence for laboratory investigation

Catheter Selection

1. For Arterial Use

– In the transfemoral approach for flush aortography (not obligatory), pig-tail catheter, 65 cm, 5 F, high-flow. In selective or superselective catheterization, cobra or sidewinder catheter with side holes, 70 cm, 5–6 F, high-flow
– In transaxillary or transbrachial catheterization, 4–5 F catheter, 100 cm

2. For Venous Use

– In transfemoral hepatic vein catheterization, cobra or sidewinder catheter with side holes, 70 cm, 5–6 F
– In transjugular or transbrachial approach, 4–5 F catheter, 100 cm
– In transhepatic portal venous catheterization, in-dwelling catheter set and cobra or headhunter catheter with side hole, 5–6 F, 70 cm

3. Guidewire Selection

– Bent-tip wire (3-mm J-wire) with moveable core, fitting catheters (150 cm) with following calibres (in inches):
0.032, 0.035, 0.038

– For superselective catheterization, Terumo guide with flexible tip, 150 cm, 0.035 in. in calibre.

4. CM Selection and Administration

CM of choice are nonionic, uroangiographic CM. In standard angiography, 76% CM are used; in intra-arterial DSA, 20%–30% CM. In both, CM is administered intraarterially. In general, only one-third as much CM is required in intraarterial DSA as in standard angiography.

For suggested flow rates of CM administered in different procedures, see (Table 9.7.1).

Complications

General Complications

These vary according to the route entry. The rate of complications rises from 1.73% for the transfemoral approach to 3.29% for transaxillary or transbrachial approach. General complications are found due to the use of CM. Local complications arise due to the puncture (bleeding, arteriovenous fistula, aneuryms), the guidewire or catheter (dissection, perforation, thrombosis) and/or compression (thrombosis, haematoma). A feared complication is the mistaken injection of CM into a lumbar artery or into the artery of Adamkiewicz (paraplegia), resulting from the selective visceral catheter coming out of the vessel during the examination (less than 1%).

Specific Complications in Percutaneous, Transhepatic Portal Venous Catherization

– Subcapsular and/or intraparenchymatous haematoma of the liver
– Puncture of the pleura with pneumothorax and/or haemothorax
– Puncture of the gallbladder with biliary peritonitis (emergency operation!)

Aftercare

The puncture site should be digitally compressed until bleeding ceases, then a compression bandage applied and the patient restricted to bed for at least 8 h. In portal venous catheterization, as in every puncture of the liver, pulse and blood pressure should be checked every half hour for 4 h.

Table 9.7.1. Administration of CM in different imaging procedures. Quantities (ml) and flow rates (ml/s)

Imaging procedure	Quantity of CM (ml)	Flow rate (ml/s)
Aorta		
SA	60	15–18
IA-DSA	15–20	10–15
Coeliac trunk		
SA	30	5–6
IA-DSA	10	5
Hepatic artery		
SA	20	4–5
IA-DSA	5–10	4–5
Splenic artery		
SA	30	4–5
IA-DSA	5–10	5
Superior mesenteric artery		
SA	50	4–5
IA-DSA	15–20	10
Transhepatic portography		
SA or IA–DSA	5–10	(by hand)
Transfemoral hepatic phlebography		
SA or IA-DSA	5–10	5–10
Indirect portography (as pharmaco-angiography)	(Prior injection of a vasodilator, e. g. 1–2 ampules of tolazoline hydrochloride [25–50 mg] dilute with 10 ml NaCl)	
Indirect mesenteric portography	(first portion, 80) 100	8–12
Indirect hepatolienography	(first portion, 60) 60	8–10

IA-DSA, intraarterial digital subtraction angiography; SA, standard angiography

Conclusions and Assessment

Angiographic procedures provide important information on the anatomy and haemodynamics of the arterial and venous system of the upper abdominal organs, especially of the portal venous system. In the sequence of procedures employed, angiographic studies are used following US, CT and MRI. Angiographic procedures are of low risk. In the abdomen, standard angiography is still justified as a routine technique not only in the GI tract but in the upper abdominal organs, too. All selective and superselective procedures, however, can also be performed as intra-arterial DSA if the patient is capable of holding his breath long enough and intestinal artefacts are not a source of disturbance.

In the liver, spleen and pancreas, angiography is indicated for preoperative clarification of vascular anatomy and for demonstrating any vascular anomalies.

In *focal lesions of the liver,* hepatic arteriography (following US, CT and radionuclide imaging with ^{99m}-Tc-HIDA) can help in diagnosing the type of haemangioma or type of focal nodular hyperplasia involved. Hepatomas based on cirrhosis are sometimes first recognized as a tumour angiographically. Vascular metastases of a carcinoid can sometimes be quantitatively better recorded by angiography than by the preceding imaging procedures.

In the *pancreas,* vascular encasement is an indication of a malignant tumour in the differentiation between pancreatitis and carcinoma of the pancreas. To locate gastrinomas, e. g. in Zollinger-Ellison syndrome, superselective intra-arterial secretin stimulation followed by angiography and simultaneous peripheral venous blood sampling to determine hormone levels is performed. The topographical correlation of the gastrin peak with the site of secretion stimulation retrospectively allows indirect localization of the gastrinoma.

In suspected insulinoma, superselective pancreatic angiography is combined with superselective pancreatic vein sampling by means of percutaneous, transhepatic, portal venous catheterization. Here also, the topographic correlation of the hormone peak (directly from the corresponding pancreatic vein sampling) with the sampling site provides the retrospective clue to insulinoma localization.

When studying the *portal venous system* in portal hypertension and for discovering perisplenic, hepatofugal flow and collateral circulation, indirect splenoportography, performed with pharma-angiography, is still the method of choice today. Direct, transfemoral, hepatic vein catheterization with hepatic venography is the method of choice for delineating a post-hepatic obstruction with hepatic vein thrombosis.

For these reasons angiographic procedures are still indispensable elements in a framework of modern imaging techniques.

9.8 Computed Tomography in the Liver, Pancreas and Spleen

A. Adam

Why?

CT is currently being challenged in certain areas by MRI but it still remains the investigation of choice for the examination of the liver, pancreas and spleen when US has failed to provide a diagnosis. It provides an overall view of the upper abdomen and this is a great advantage as diseases affecting one of these three organs frequently present with secondary abnormalities in the other two. For example, pancreatic carcinoma may be associated with hepatic and, occasionally, splenic metastases. Another example is cirrhosis of the liver due to chronic alcoholism which may be associated with pancreatitis and splenic varices.

Another advantage of CT scanning is that following administration of CM it can provide important information about the vascularity of the organs being examined. The viable parts of the pancreas following a severe attack of pancreatitis can be identified and hepatic or splenic infarction can be demonstrated.

The exquisite contrast sensitivity of CT and its ability to measure X-ray attenuation accurately can provide diagnostic information such as the occurrence of haemorrhage in a pancreatic pseudocyst and can demonstrate minute amounts of calcification in the pancreas in the cases of chronic pancreatitis.

When?

CT has become widely available in recent years and a routine examination following the injection of intravenous CM is indicated when an US study has not provided a diagnosis. MRI is challenging CT, especially in the investigation of liver diseases, but the speed and convenience of CT and the ease with which interventional procedures can be performed, combined with its more widespread availability, make it preferable to MRI in most centres.

More invasive studies, such as CT arteriography (CTA), CT-arterioportography (CTAP) and CT following hepatic intra-arterial Lipiodol (HIAL) are usually reserved for patients with primary or metastatic liver tumors being considered for partial hepatic resection. These studies are usually considered as the definitive investigations of such patients and are performed when all other examinations, including angiography, have not demonstrated a lesion in the part of the liver which is to be preserved at surgery.

Which Contrast Medium?

Dynamic CT scanning, CTA, CTAP and delayed CT scanning are performed using water-soluble, iodinated CM. Although small differences have been demonstrated in the rate of diffusion of CM into the hepatic parenchyma, the magnitude of these differences is not such as to affect the choice of CM in practice. In making the selection, the principles applied are those which govern the choice of CM for intravascular use in general.

Nevertheless one point which must be considered specifically is the volume and rate of injection of the CM employed for dynamic CT studies of the liver: a 50-g iodine dose is often given as 180 ml of 60% CM. It is well known that patients with normal cardiac function can tolerate an acute intravascular volume expansion of 1 l. The volume of 180 ml of 60% ionic

CM is equivalent to 750 ml/l of normal saline. This volume load of CM has been accepted as safe in adquately hydrated patients with normal cardio-renal function who undergo angiographic procedures. The only difference between the method of CM delivery employed in angiography (3 ml kg bw/h) and the technique usually employed in CT is that the CM is delivered over 2 min with due regard for the patient's cardiac function. Nonionic CM, which has approximately half the osmolality of ionic CM, can be used as an alternative for patients with abnormal cardiac function. In patients with normal baseline serum creatinine levels there is no abnormal elevation of serum creatinine at 24, 48 and 72 h after the procedure. In patients with serum creatinine levels greater than 1.5 mg/dl (132.6 μmol/l), a non-con-trast-enhanced CT scan should be obtained. If results from the non-contrast-enhanced CT scan are negative in a patient with clinically suspected liver metastases, the use of MRI should be considered.

Lipiodol injected selectively into the hepatic artery is taken up by tumours in a variety of patterns. Normal hepatic parenchyma also takes up the Lipiodol, but the CM is cleared from normal liver within approximately 1 week, whereas it is retained in tumours. In general, vascular tumours such as hepatomas take up Lipiodol in a diffuse manner, whereas avascular lesions may not retain it at all or may demonstrate uptake only around the periphery of the lesion. It is thought that Lipiodol is taken up by tumours due to some abnormality of neoplastic vasculature which encourages leak-age of CM into the tumour. Another explanation is that Kupffer cells clear Lipiodol from the normal hepatic parenchyma but as such cells do not exist within neoplastic tissue Lipiodol is retained within the latter. Usually ap-proximately 10 ml Lipiodol emulsion is injected into the hepatic artery and the CT scan is performed 7–10 days later but both the contrast volume and the timing of the examination vary considerably from centre to centre.

Promising results have been obtained in recent years with intravenously administered emulsified oily CM. These have been taken up by the liver parenchyma and focal lesions appear as low attenuation masses within the opacified hepatic parenchyma on CT. Several such agents have been tried over the years but most of them have proved too hepatotoxic for clinical use. A new agent, Intraiodol, which was developed in Sweden appears to be less toxic than previous agents but has been used only in a small number of patients to date on an experimental basis.

Which Method?

The Spleen

Specific examinations of the spleen by CT scanning are rarely performed and the organ is usually inspected when a study of the liver is done, in which case the volume of contrast and timing of scans is determined by the type of liver study being performed. Nevertheless when splenic lesions are being sought specifically it is best to administer approximately 180 ml of 60% CM as described below for dynamic liver CT but to delay scanning until 90–120 s after the beginning of the injection. This is because scans performed soon after the injection of CM are likely to show patchy areas of unequal attenuation due to differential flow patterns in the red and white splenic pulp. Later on, equalization of splenic parenchymal opacification increases the likelihood of lesions being detected and reduces the number of false-positive and false-negative results.

The Pancreas

Dynamic CT scanning is the method of choice for the routine examination of the pancreas. Some 150 ml of CM can be injected in a biphasic technique: 50 ml is given as 5 ml/s for 10 s followed by 1 ml/s for 100 s. Magnified contiguous sections of the pancreas are obtained every 4 or 5 min. It is best to use a dedicated CT volume flow rate injector that can be operated by a radiographer from the CT console. Contrast given by hand injection is not as accurate in its timing, not as reproducible and not as convenient. With a volume flow rate injector, CM is delivered through standard venous cannulae (19 or 20 gauge) either 1 1/4 in (3.2 cm) or 2 in (5.1 cm) in length preferably into antecubital veins. The radiologist must palpate the injection site to ensure that the CM delivered through the plastic venous cannula does not extravasate. If extravasation occurs, the injection should be stopped immediately. The optimal method for delivering CM through antecubital veins is to position the patient's arm at a right angle to the chest by placing the palm of the hand against the face of the CT gantry. This ensures that injected CM is not constricted at the thoracic outlet. Unlike the liver, which is mainly supplied by the portal vein, the pancreas has an arterial blood supply and the pancreatic parenchyma enhances earlier than the liver. Scanning should start 15–20 s after the beginning of the injection of CM. Almost all examinations will be completed in under 2 min, well within the period of excellent opacification of the pancreas.

Dynamic CT of the pancreas is a very accurate way of establishing the presence of vascular encasement by malignant tumours and demonstrating the extent of pancreatic neoplasms. In most centres three or four scans are performed during held inspiration. Then the patient takes another breath and the procedure is repeated until the whole organ has been scanned.

With the advent of faster CT scanners with tubes of greater heat capacity it has become possible to scan the pancreas very fast while the patient breathes quietly. As a bolus 100 ml CM is administered by hand and scanning begins immediately after the end of the injection. Scans obtained using this method may demonstrate some respiratory movement artefacts but if a scanner capable of 2-s scans and a 3.5- to 5-s interscan delay is used, the artefact is minimal and does not affect the diagnostic quality of the examination, which is fully equivalent to that of CT scans obtained using the conventional technique described above. There are several advantages to this approach: a smaller volume of CM is used, the volume flow rate injector is unnecessary and the examination is completed in less time than with the conventional method – usually in less than 90 s. In addition the fact that the patient is allowed to breath during the examination has obvious advantages with elderly patients and those with respiratory aliments who may find it difficult to suspend respiration.

Very occasionally CT arteriography is useful for the demonstration of vascular neoplasms of the pancreas. A catheter is inserted selectively into the coeliac axis and 60% CM is injected at 1 ml/s for 50 s. Dynamic scanning with incremental table movement is used to examine the whole organ. Scanning begins immediately after the start of the injection. Vascular lesions such as insulinomas are shown as hyperattenuating masses.

The Liver

Dynamic Hepatic CT. It is best to use a volume flow rate injector as described above for pancreatic CT. Some 180 ml of 60% CM is used at 5 ml/s for 10 s and 1 ml/s for 130 s. Scanning with incremental table movement begins 40 s after the start of the injection and continues until the whole of the liver has been examined. The normal liver is supplied 75% from the portal vein and 25% from the hepatic artery, while metastases receive virtually 100% of their blood supply from the hepatic artery. Hepatic parenchymal enhancement reaches a plateau approximately 40 s after a bolus injection of CM. Most metastases are hypovascular and appear as low attenuation lesions within the opacified parenchyma. Tumours that may be hypervascular in relation to normal hepatic parenchyma (e.g. primary hepatoma and metastases from pancreatis islet cell tumour, carcinoid, and renal cell carcinoma) may be isodense during an incremental dynamic CT obtained during bolus contrast administration, whereas a 40-s delay after the beginning of the injection reduces the likelihood of such lesions being isodense with the liver parenchyma. Nevertheless patients with suspected hypervascular tumours should have both a non-contrast and a dynamic post-contrast study.

CM delivered as described above ensures positive enhancement of the hepatic veins in addition to the portal veins, so that detected lesions can be located with respect to specific hepatic lobes and segments. Hepatic CT usually requires 12–20 contiguous sections (average, 16) and can be achieved in less than 2 min after the beginning of scanning in almost all patients when using a modern fast CT scanner.

Unfortunately in many centres infusion techniques are still used in CT of the liver. With these methods significant portions of the liver may not be examined until 5–10 min after the beginning of the CM infusion. This may result in metastases being isodense in the normal liver. In other cases the increase in attenuation of the hepatic parenchyma may be insufficient to reveal small lesions. Dynamic CT of the liver as described above should be the routine method of scanning this organ. If a volume flow rate injector is not available, hand injection of a bolus of CM followed by dynamic scanning is still better than an infusion technique.

Compared with unenhanced CT, use of dynamic sequential hepatic CT does not markedly increase the number of patients correctly diagnosed as having liver metastases, but the number of lesions detected can be increased by as much as 40% and this is a most important consideration for patients being considered for partial hepatic resection.

Delayed Hepatic CT. Delayed hepatic CT is a technique that uses CM contained within the interstitial spaces of the liver and within hepatocytes 4–6 h after the initial injection. This represents the small percentage of CM "vicariously" taken up and excreted by the liver, as well as CM that remains in equilibrium with that circulating intravascularly. Provided that an adequate iodine load, at least 60 g, has been used initially, a 20 Hounsfield unit (HU) elevation of hepatic CT number is seen at 4–6 h. The CM is administered intravenously and as the examination is not performed until much later the injection can be given quite slowly.

Delayed hepatic CT is a very sensitive technique in the detection of hepatic metastases and has a lower false-positive rate than CTAP. Nevertheless, few centres use this method routinely mainly because it is inconvenient to schedule patients to be examined 4–6 h after the initial injection of CM.

CT Arteriography. Hepatic artery CTA is performed following selective hepatic arteriography. The arteriogram is obtained to define vascular anatomy for the surgeon, as well as to detect additional hepatic lesions. If the hepatic tumour appears to be resectable at the completion of arteriography, the catheter is left in the hepatic artery and the patient is transferred to the CT scanner. The liver is then scanned using automatic table incrementation, 10-mm contiguous scans and the dynamic mode of the machine. A cluster of three of four scans is obtained followed by a 10-s intergroup delay, to allow for patient respiration. During scanning 30% CM is infused through the hepatic artery at the rate of 1 ml/s. Approximately 100 ml CM is required for most patients. Thus, the additional iodine load to the patient is only minimal and is usually quite safe.

Hepatic artery CTA has been shown to be more sensitive than incremental dynamic CT for specific lesion detection. Approximately 30%–55% of patients will have additional lesions detected.

A significant proportion of patients will have accessory hepatic arteries which must be catheterized, otherwise lesions supplied by those arteries will be missed. Those metastases receive virtually all their blood supply from the hepatic artery, unlike the normal hepatic parenchyma, which is supplied by both the hepatic artery and portal vein. CTA identifies metastases as hyperattenuated in relation to background hepatic parenchyma. Vascular lesions are easier to visualize on CTA than relatively avascular tumours. One of the pitfalls of hepatic CTA is that layering or unusual flow patterns may result in the liver. These patterns correspond to main or subsegmental branches of the hepatic artery, which are more or less opacified. Hepatic contrast differences result primarily as a result of flow going to one portion of the liver through the catheter, while the adjacent portion of the liver does not receive CM and thus is not opacified.

CT Arterioportography. In CTAP, CM is injected selectively into the superior mesenteric artery at 2–3 ml/s for a total of 100–150 ml, using a volume flow rate injector. The liver is imaged 30 s after the beginning of CM injection. CTAP is a "super" intravenous bolus contrast-enhanced CT study in which the injected CM is delivered selectively into the portal venous supply without distribution to and dilution with the central blood volume. This results in greater hepatic parenchymal enhancement and contrast differentiation between focal lesions and background. CTAP is easier to implement than hepatic artery injection CT because the catheter tip needs only to be placed in the superior mesenteric artery distal to any anomalous hepatic artery branches. Parenchymal enchancement of 80–100 HU can be achieved, compared with parenchymal enchancement of 50–70 HU achieved with intravenous bolus injection.

Perfusion defects may be observed due to incomplete admixture of enhanced blood in the superior mesenteric vein with unenhanced blood in the splenic vein, resulting in hypoperfusion of the left hepatic lobe. In addition, central metastases may compress central portal vein branches, resulting in hypoperfusion defects. Although nontumorous attenuation differences are significantly more frequent with CTAP than with dynamic CT, they are seldom a diagnostic problem because of their geographic pattern. In patients in whom it is unclear whether a hypoperfusion defect or a true focal lesion exists, it is advisable to perform a delayed hepatic CT study 4–6 h after CTAP. However, lesions may be missed in areas which have not opacified sufficiently and it is important not to interpret CTAP in isolation from a conventional dynamic study and, if necessary, other examinations such as US and MRI.

What Are the Complications of these Procedures?

All methods of CT which utilize iodinated CM may be associated with hypersensitivity reactions and with disturbances of renal or cardiovascular function or with clotting disorders, pyrexias and other rarer reactions which are described elsewhere in this book. CT arteriography, CT arterioportography and Lipiodol CT may also be associated with the various complications of angiography described in the relevant chapters.

Patient tolerance of hepatic intra-arterial Lipiodol CT is usually excellent in cases of selective hepatic artery injection. Occasionally, nonselective injection into the coeliac axis is utilized and this sometimes results in certain side effects immediately after the injection: approximately one-third of patients experience nausea or vomiting which regresses spontaneously in 15–20 min. In patients with an accessory hepatic artery arising from the superior mesenteric artery, an attempt to inject Lipiodol selectively into the accessory hepatic branch may result in a reflux of Lipiodol into the superior mesenteric artery. In such patients diarrhoea may be observed for approximately 6 h but tends to resolve without sequelae. Acute cholecystitis requiring cholecystectomy has been described following hepatic artery injection of Lipiodol.

Conclusions

In the investigation of the liver, spleen and pancreas dynamic CT following the intravenous injection of CM should follow US scanning when the latter has failed to provide a diagnosis. In patients being considered for partial hepatic resection in whom dynamic CT has not revealed any lesions in the part ot the liver which is to be preserved, CTAP is probably the investigation of choice. If this procedure reveals definite lesions, surgery is contraindicated. If very small lesions of questionable significance are detected, it is best to proceed to surgery and confirm the presence of such lesions with peroperative US rather than deny the patient the chance of a cure.

9.9   The Gastrointestinal Tract

W. Dihlmann and *L. Hering*

Why?

The primary goal of contrast radiology of the gastrointestinal (GI) tract is to produce the most *selective* visualization of the digestive tract possible. The CM suspension coats the inner surface of the digestive tract as a thin film, making it possible to detect or exclude lesions. Contrast-enhanced images can also provide morphological and functional information by presenting a cast of the digestive tract or, on the basis of its incompressibility, allow detailed views of the tract's macromorphology. These contrast examinations may be classified by technique as: mucosal relief, double contrast, distension and compression. They may be used, depending the anatomy, topography and the problem being clinically investigated, as complementary, alternative or essential examinations.

X-ray study of the GI tract is a noninvasive imaging technique. In most cases results, in good hands, are comparable to those of endoscopy.

When?

Imaging of the GI tract is indicated for the detection of lesions, such as erosions, ulcers, perforations, hernias, varices and tumours, and to clarify morphological and functional changes. It may be further indicated in postoperative monitoring of symptoms such as nausea, vomiting, bleeding, or persistent diarrhoea with signs of malabsorption and colicky abdominal pain.

Owing to the similar densities of organs and tissues surrounding the GI tract, CM is essential. The GI tract can be imaged in whole or in part, as required, and there is great variation in examination technique and the type, concentration and amount of CM used.

Contrast Media in the X-Ray Examination of the Hypopharynx and Oesophagus

Although there are certain advantages to the use of barium pastes and other special CM preparations whose passage through the oesophagus may be observed they do not actually produce any convincing additional understanding of oesophageal morphology and function. Thus, in practice, those barium CM used for visualizing stomach and duodenum are also employed in the imaging of the oesophagus.

In clinical dysphagia, and particularly in cases of suspected aspiration of a foreign body, an absorbable, water-soluble, iodinated CM (if possible low osmolar and nonionic) or Gastrografin or Peritrast Oral GI (diluted until isotonic) should be used in place of a barium suspension. Barium CM are further contraindicated if there is a question of oesophageal perforation, e.g. after cauterization, endoscopy, or endoscopic intervention, or if atresias or other congenital or acquired fistulae are to be excluded.

By sipping the barium CM the morphology and function of the hypopharynx and oesophagus, their fold pattern and tone can be evaluated. Examination of the gastro-oesophageal junction is, however, part of every such examination of the oesophagus. Thus, even if only the oesophagus is to be imaged the patient should have an empty stomach in order to obtain precise information about this region (hiatal hernia, reflux, reflux effects).

With segmental double-contrast studies of the oesophagus small, minimal changes (especially those arising from early cancer) and erosions and flat ulcers can be seen. The intravenous injection of a parasympatholytic is advisable, e.g. Buscopan (hyoscine butylbromide) 20(–40) mg according to body weight, in order to produce oesophageal hypotonia. After a short pause, a high-density barium suspension should then be drunk. Swallowing air or drinking tap water immediately thereafter produces the double-contrast: the patient holds the cup with the barium CM in one hand and the cup with tap water in the other and drinks according to the radiologist's directions. The double-contrast examination is performed with the fluoroscopic table tilted at about a 45° angle.

"Retrograde" double-contrast visualization of the oesophagus is performed with the patient standing. He takes the CO_2-releasing additive into his mouth and washes it down with a few milliliters of water or with a sip of CM suspension. Then he swallows additional barium suspension under fluoroscopic control. The examiner waits for regurgitation of gas and then exposes X-ray films.

Examination for submucosal oesophageal varices in the tubular oesophageal segment is performed with the patient in supine position (possibly slightly tilted, head down). In order to examine a nonphysiological gastro-oesophageal reflux, it is advisable also to examine the patient in a prone position (with slightly raised left side of the body) and to increase the intra-abdominal pressure by placing a 10- to 20-cm-thick compression pillow between the table and the patient's upper midabdomen.

According to the literature radiological examination alone is not always sufficient to be able to confirm or exclude reflux oesophagitis. Endoscopy or endoscopic biopsies are better in this case; this is also true in infants, children and adolescents [11].

Contrast Media in the X-Ray Examination of the Stomach and Duodenum

Barium Sulphate

In comparison to the thoracic and abdominal soft tissues, barium has a relatively high atomic number of 56. Moreover, the form in which it is generally used, barium sulphuricum purissimum (German Pharmacopoeia, 9th edn.; European Pharmacopoeia), is difficult to dissolve in water, is osmotically inactive and causes no chemical or biochemical reactions in the GI tract. Thus, barium is not absorbed in the alimentary canal and, consequently, systematic barium toxicity does not develop. A barium sulphate CM suspension has to be of high quality and has to be ingested in sufficient quantity, ca. 150–250 ml.

Due to its high density, barium absorbs a larger portion of the X-radiation than body soft tissues and provides a positive contrast effect.

The following are specifications for barium sulphate suspensions. The barium sulphate content mut be at least 1 g/ml. Thus, in preparing barium sulphate in powder form, barium density must also be considered. The diameter of the barium particles should be about 1 μm and the suspension should be of a creamy consistency to achieve an appropriate viscosity. Thus, in summary, a barium CM suspension for the barium meal must possess low viscosity combined with high barium sulphate content.

Colloidal additives stabilize the suspension to militate against formation of aggregates or bubbles, i.e. agglomeration and sedimentation tendencies are inhibited. Moreover, such organic additives prevent "tearing" of the CM film which forms on the mucosal surface. The taste of the suspension must not influence gastric secretion. A CM suspension of this quality is characterized by its ability to adhere well to the inner surface of the stomach and duodenum, to form an even mucosal coating, and, even as a thin layer at X-ray tube voltages of ca. 100 kV, to provide good contrast.

CM suspensions are non-Newtonian fluids [15]. Their viscosity thus diminishes with increasing shear rates. This thixotropy can be measured in a rotation viscometer as a function of revolutions per minute (rpm) and may be expressed in centipoise (cP; poise is the unit of dynamic viscosity).

The double-contrast technique (see below) has led to an improvement in CM quality, but at the same time, the underlying idea of the double-contrast technique is based on certain physical properties of *barium CM*. The so-called *high-density (HD) CM,* e.g. Micropaque Oral HD or E-Z-HD, both possess the appropriate characteristics:

1. The weight-volume ratio is ca. 2 g/ml and is thus relatively high.
2. In the commercial, high-density CM, particle mixtures with diameters of 2–20 μm are found and it is desirable to have the highest possible proportion of larger barium-sulphate particles.
3. Viscosity does not exceed 100 cP [21].

If a barium CM satisfies these conditions it is termed a high-density CM; in the double-contrast examination of the stomach and duodenum under conditions of pharmacological hypotonia (see below), it manifests the following behaviour:

The particle size and greater density of high-density CM guarantee that a ~ 1-mm-thin, nontearing CM film, sufficient to absorb X-rays, follows the contours of the mucous membrane and clearly defines them. (Standard barium CM result in a 2- to 5-mm thick mucosal coating, sometimes concealing the contours of the gastric mucous membrane.) High-density CM are also viscous enough to stick to small (pathological) protrusions.

One can conclude from the physical characteristics of barium CM as a non-Newtonian solution (see above) that the secret of double-contrast examinations of the stomach and duodenum is to rotate the patient around his long axis. In so doing the CM becomes thinner and runnier than in a motionless patient. In this way, it is easier for the CM to enter the tiny mucosal recesses making up the areae gastricae. In contrast, in a resting position, viscosity increases and the thus thicker CM adheres better to small (pathological) mucosal protrusions.

High-density CM sediment faster than (standard) non-high-density barium sulphate suspensions. In relatively rapid gastroduodenal transit (GDT), this does not disturb the examination; however, CM suspensions with a barium content of greater than 1.5 g/ml are no longer suitable for the longer examinations of the small intestine [21].

Iodinated X-Ray Contrast Media

Water-soluble, iodinated CM are also "positive" CM and have recognized indications in radiological examinations of the intestinal tract, mainly to avoid the side effects of barium sulphate. The primary indications for their *oral* use include: detection and localization of a clinically suspected wall perforation, detection of postoperative suture leak and, GI transit in known cases of colonic stenosis and as a general rule in the presence of symptoms of ileus. Due to their relatively poor adhesiveness to the gastric mucosa they are not very suitable for visualizing circumscribed (flat) gastric lesions.

The CM for oral (and rectal) administration currently available contain 300–400 mg I/ml. A tri-iodinated organic acid salt such as, for example, meglumine diatrizoate, provides X-ray absorption and positive contrast.

For these CM, only small amounts, i.e. less than 5% of the administered dose is absorbed from the GI and excreted via the kidneys in 24 h. The kidneys also excrete *all* the CM that leaves the intestine because of inflammation perforation or wound dehiscence. The secondary contrast imaging of the kidneys is, therefore, an indirect sign of contrast leakage, ca. 30–60 min after CM administration.

Dilute barium sulphate suspensions and dilute preparations of water-soluble, iodinated, GI CM are both used in contrast-enhanced abdominal CT. They are available from the producer either in ready-to-use form or are accompanied by recommendations for dilution.

Gaseous Contrast Media

Gaseous CM, such as air or CO_2, absorb and scatter X-rays more weakly than body tissue, thus producing a negative contrast effect. Commercially available CO_2-releasing additives increase gas pressure in the gut and are used in conjunction with positive CM for double-contrast examinations. By adding an organic despumator, the formation of tiny bubbles that would otherwise interfere is inhibited.

Examination Techniques

GI transit is assessed using the techniques of distension and mucosal relief, compression (manually in a radiation-shielding glove or by means of a compression tube) and double contrast.

Distension. The contours of the stomach and the duodenal cap are examined in distension and the tone and swallowing mechanisms are observed. Moreover, it is distension that provides the primary image of the form of the stomach and duodenum and conveys information about their positional relationships with respect to other abdominal organs. This is an indisputable advantage over endoscopy.

Mucosal Relief. The height and width (normally 4–5 mm) of the mucosal folds depend on, among other things, on the fluid content of the submucosa and upon the state of contraction of the muscle layers. The term "mucosal folds" is not strictly correct, since both mucosa and submucosa are involved in forming these folds. The relief of the stomach mucosa produced by these folds can be visualized by partly filling the stomach or parts of the stomach, where the CM collects only in the depressions between the folds. In the study of stomach mucosal relief, those changes of the inner gastric surface that at least exceed the scale of the folds can be recognized [22].

Compression. In compression, the relief of the compressed part of the stomach is initially revealed and can be evaluated. In the stomach and the duodenal cap, the image of the folds vanishes as compression continues. In the pylorus and in the still compressible part of the body, fine detail then becomes visible. The "areae gastricae" form the anatomical substrate of fine relief. They can be recognized as a round, oval or polygonal net-like structure, with maximum diameters of 3–4 mm and are real anatomical entities. However, they are not always radiologically visible.

In compression, raised lesions are seen as recesses and depressed lesions as circumscribed collections of the meal.

Double Contrast. In general, this term denotes the simultaneous use of "positive" and "negative" CM in the visualization of objects such as hollow organs and joint cavities. After administering a "positive" CM and manoeuvring the patient to coat the wall position gas, or some other "negative" CM is introduced and the anatomical features of the mucosa may be well displayed.

There are three different routes to obtaining "negative" contrast:
1. Shifting the physiological air bubbles from one part of the stomach to the other by changing the patient's position
2. Insufflation via a stomach tube
3. Administering a CO_2-releasing additive.

In the visualization of the stomach and duodenum it is useful to inject spasmolytics to reduce motility and thus the emptying of the stomach and duodenum and to allow distension. Glucagon, the polypeptide secreted by the alpha cells of the pancreas, and Buscopan (hyoscine butylbromide), a synthetic parasympatholytic (20–40 mg i.v.), are frequently administered to induce pharmacological hypotonia and hypomotility.

Thus, the double-contrast technique requires specific positive CM, a sufficient quantity of "negative" CM, and artificial hypotonia and hypomotility.

With this technique even slight differences in the level of the inner surface of the stomach and duodenum are made visible. And by turning the patient from his right side to his left side and then back, the CM fluctuates between the pylorus and the fundus. At the same time, the air or air-carbon dioxide mix moves in the opposite direction, providing the desired double contrast. The effect of frequent rotation of the patient around his long axis was discussed earlier.

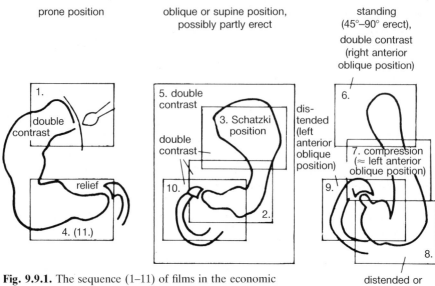

Fig. 9.9.1. The sequence (1–11) of films in the economic standardized X-ray examination of the stomach (see text)

The frequency with which a radiological examination of the stomach and duodenum performed in double contrast successfully images the areae gastricae and complete (varioliform) gastric erosions is held to be the *criterion of the biological quality* of this procedure [14].

The general technique of radiological examination of the stomach and duodenum [4] as well as of several of its variations in particular situations are dealt with comprehensively in the literature [3, 14, 21].

The X-Ray Examination of the Small Intestine

Diseases of the small intestine are most frequently found in the duodenum and the terminal ileum. However, the small intestine as a whole can also be affected.

In radiological examinations of the stomach the duodenum is examined as well. These two structures are also very accessible to endoscopy. However, the complete examination of the small intestine remains the domain of the radiologist and currently a standardized double-contrast procedure modified according to Sellink termed enteroclysis (Fig. 9.9.1) is performed.

Radiological examination of the small intestine is absolutely contraindicated in the case of colonic obstruction or gut perforation.

Preparatory purgative measures are required in order to ensure the unhindered passage of CM. Residual stool in the intestine creates mechanical obstacles and may lead to misinterpretation.

Enteroclysis

Enteroclysis requires the introduction of a (reusable) catheter. Common catheter types for use in the small bowel are 130–150 cm long, have a lumen of 2.5–3 mm and they contain a flexible inner guide-wire.

After local anaesthesia, the catheter is introduced transnasally or transorally, guided through the oesophagus and stomach and through and beyond the pylorus up to the duodenal flexure. There are various ways of surmounting possible difficulties connected with the placement of the catheter. These include the repositioning of the patient, e.g. sitting him up or manoeuvering him onto his right or left side. Air insufflation through the catheter when it reaches the prepyloric region to dilate the pylorus is also useful. The supplementary administration of metoclopramide promotes motility and the transport of the catheter tip. The intermittent use of the guidewire plays an important role in the placement of the probe, in order, for example, to stop the catheter from unwinding in the stomach or the tip from springing back out of the duodenum. Test CM administration is helpful in localizing the catheter tip on occasion.

Contrast Media in the X-Ray Examination of the Small Intestine

For the double-contrast X-ray examination of the small intestine, a thin barium suspension is required [20]. For example, the mixture of one part Micropaque Liquid (barium sulphate) and two parts water, e.g. ca. 300 ml Micropaque and 600 ml water, has proven effective. It is advisable to warm the CM suspension close to body temperature before use. For double contrast, methylcellulose is used in a 0.5% aqueous solution [2], for example, 10 g methylcellulose to which 2 l of water is slowly added under constant stirring. Lump formation must be avoided.

Here, the barium sulphate suspension represents the "positive" and the methylcellulose the "negative" CM. The barium sulphate suspension ensures that the wall is coated evenly, whereas methylcellulose is both a distension medium for the hollow organ and a provider of double contrast.

Instillation of Double-Contrast Agent

After the catheter has been positioned in the duodenal flexure, the CM is infused. An even CM flow rate of 75 ml/min has been shown to be effective. On average, 500 ml CM suspension is administered via the catheter.

Then the methylcellulose solution is instilled. This pushes the CM bolus forward from behind and provides the desired double contrast. The flow rate of methylcellulose usually lies between 100 and 200 ml/min. About 800 ml (500–1500 ml) is required for enteroclysis.

In order to maintain a constant flow rate of CM and methylcellulose, commercially available pumps should be used. Alternatively, a large-volume syringe or an infusion bottle suspended from a tripod can be used for manual injection.

Small-intestine motility should be taken into account in determining the best instillation rate for an individual patient. A lower rate of about 50 ml/min must be used, for example, when there is danger of reflux (in the stomach) and reduced motility in the upper jejunum. A higher barium suspension flow rate of about 100 ml/min is advisable in accelerated intestinal passage in order to ensure even and sufficient contrast imaging of all segments of the small intestine.

The X-Ray Examination of the Colon

The double-contrast technique is currently used in radiological examinations of the colon. It offers a diagnostic overview of the entire colon (Fig. 9.9.2).

Indications for such an examination range from the exclusion of stenotic lesions in the abdomen to the detection of a malignant or benign colonic or rectal tumour, diverticulosis and inflammatory disease of the colon.

Intestinal perforation and toxic megacolon count as *contraindications* for double-contrast examination of the colon.

Relative contraindications of double-contrast examinations include poor general state of health (including cardiac and respiratory insufficiency); acute ulcerative colitis; stenotic or perforating diverticulitis; recent surgery, biopsy or polypectomy; and incontinence of the anal sphincter muscles.

Before beginning the X-ray examination, the following precautionary measures should be taken:
1. The examination should begin with digital examination of the rectum.
2. To avoid perforation, rectal balloon catheters should not be used.
3. A safety interval of 2–3 weeks should be observed following a biopsy or polypectomy.
4. The introduction of CM should take place under fluoroscopic control.
5. In cases of obstruction, and if the patient complains of pain on bowel distension, the CM enema must not be forcibly continued.

A complete cleansing of the colon is essential for a successful X-ray examination. Residual stool obstructs passage of the CM and limits the diagnostic usefulness of the procedure. Options for preparatory cleansing of the colon should be judged in terms of their practicality, the time they require, whether the patient can be expected to tolerate the procedure and how thorough they are.

To relax the colon, and so that the barium sulphate suspension adheres better to the intestinal mucosa, an anticholinergic agent is given (1 mg atropine sulphate orally) 30 min before examination. Glaucoma patients should receive instead 1 mg glucagon intravenously prior to administration of the CM enema.

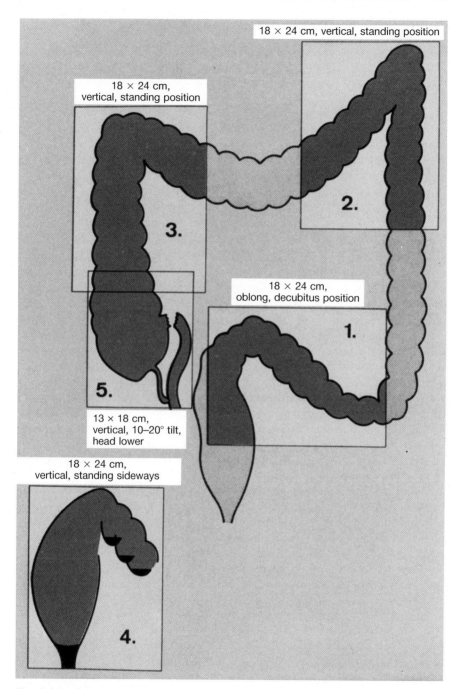

Fig. 9.9.2. Colon contrast enema in double contrast. Minimal series of X-ray films produced under fluoroscopic control (nrs. 1–5 from [5])

Contrast Media in the X-Ray Examination of the Colon

Stable barium sulphate suspension containing ca. 50–65 mg barium sulphate/ml (such as Barotrast or Micropaque Colon) that demonstrate good wall adhesiveness to the intestinal mucosa are the CM used in double-contrast examination of the colon. These are thinner than the suspensions used in gastroduodenal examinations.

If the aim of the examination is to localize a mechanical obstruction of the colon preoperatively or if intussusception is suspected, double-contrast examination of the colon with a barium sulphate suspension is strictly contraindicated. In such cases, a water-soluble, iodinated CM should be used.

Examination Techniques

During the introduction of the rectal tube used for CM administration, the patient lies in the left lateral position. The barium CM suspension should be warmed to body temperature and be free of air bubbles. The patient then turns to the prone position. The examiner observes the CM flow fluoroscopically for a short period. While doing this, he tilts the patient slightly, head down. Alternately moving the patient laterally to the left and to the right in accordance with intestinal turns assists CM flow into the body. When the CM reaches the hepatic flexure of the colon, CM administration is stopped. After the rectal tube is removed, the patient goes to the toilet to empty his CM-filled bowels. The defecatory compression of the abdomen pushes the CM into the caecum – usually without CM entry into the terminal ileum. If such is desired, however, in suspected terminal ileitis or ulcerative colitis enema administration is continued until the CM enters the ascending colon.

After the bowels are emptied, the examiner reintroduces the rectal tube. In order to achieve double contrast, a sufficient amount of air is insufflated as negative CM (1800–2000 ml).

After air insufflation into the rectum and sigmoid colon, the first films of the sigmoid are produced before the images are overlapped by retrograde contrast filling the ileum. After ample air insufflation and dilation of the intestine, the patient should be turned around his long axis at least twice in order to ensure an even contrast coating of all intestinal segments.

A complete overview of the entire colon can be obtained with eight standard X-rays. Some authors take as few as six X-rays for "colon status" [1], whereas others require 10–14 films [16, 23].

The author [5] has described an approach to the examination yielding complete visualization at reasonable cost and with the lowest possible radiation exposure (Fig. 9.9.3).

Side Effects of Barium Sulphate Suspension

In constipation-prone patients, there may be a longer transit time for orally administered CM and the barium sulphate may clump due to increased

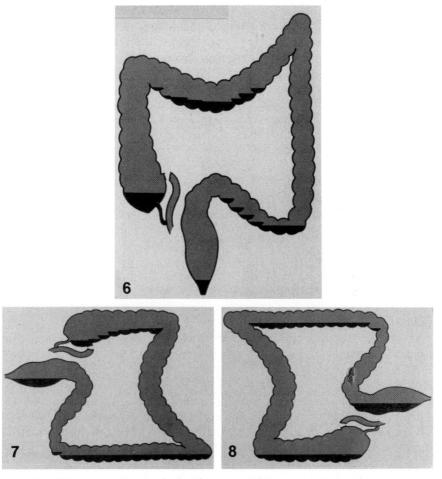

Fig. 9.9.3. Colon contrast enema in double contrast, three survey X-rays of the colon on a grid wall tripod (6–8, 35 × 43 cm film format, vertical format for standing position, oblong format for left and right lateral position)

fluid absorption. It is advisable in these cases to administer laxatives after gastroduodenal X-ray examination.

Harmful effects are to be expected if barium sulphate penetrates into the soft tissues of the neck, mediastinum, peritoneal cavity or into the retroperitoneal space through a perforation of the GI tract. The barium sulphate induces a typical tissue reaction outside the intestine. Initially, inflammation develops with exudation and leucocytic phagocytosis of the barium particles. Within a few hours, the barium sulphate has been enveloped to such a great extent by fibrin that it can no longer be washed out. Foreign-body granulomata and fibrosis ensue. On the one hand, this fibrosis results in the encapsulation of the barium sulphate; on the other, such massive fibrosis promotes degeneration in the peritoneal cavity and adhesions of the two lining membranes. Even years after barium CM has penetrated into extraintestinal spaces, episodes of ileus and even ureteric obstruction can occur as a result of scar tissue contraction. In the mediastinum, oesophageal obstruction and compromise of venous drainage may develop as late complications.

In such cases the acute prognosis is poor if bacteria contaminate the leaking CM. In particular, faecal contamination is cause for great concern. Barium sulphate rarely escapes into the veins of portal circulation unless the intestinal wall has been breached and there has been a lengthy transit time, for example due to stenosis.

Dysphagia can lead to the aspiration of barium sulphate. It is usually expelled by coughing. In older patients or those persons in poor general health, however, fatalities due to pneumonia and septicaemia have been described after barium-sulphate aspiration.

Side Effects of Water-Soluble, Iodinated Contrast Media

Water-soluble iodinated CM for the X-ray examination of the GI are well tolerated but side effects that the practising physician must be aware of do occur.

Prolonged *localized* CM retention behind stenoses of obstructions, for example, can induce mucosal irritation, erosions and necrosis with a risk of bleeding.

Water-soluble, ionic, iodinated CM for the GI tract have strong osmotic effects. Their osmolality can be six times higher than that of blood plasma. This is the source of their laxative effect: the fluid shifts from the blood into the intestinal lumen stimulate the stretch receptors of the intestinal wall, and increase motility. Moreover, it has been deduced from animal experiments that CM-induced release of the biogenic amine serotonin directly stimulates the smooth muscle of the intestinal wall [18].

As a rule, CM manufacturers suggest maximum doses per examination for their preparations so as to avoid hypovolemia and electrolyte disturbances in dehydrated patients, accompanied sometimes by adverse effects on the cardiovascular system. Especially in old, severely ill patients in poor general health, but also in the newborn, infants and small children, the possibility of such side effects of iodinated GI CM has to be considered.

In patients with dysphagia, the aspiration of larger amounts of CM can lead to intra-alveolar pulmonary oedema and to pneumonia, in part as a result of the osmotic effects of CM. In spite of the low absorption rates of water-soluble iodinated CM (see above), CM allergic or hypersensitivity reactions can occur. Caution is advisable in patients with (latent and manifest) hyperthyroidism.

In order to avoid the hyperosmolality complications in at-risk patients, it is advisable to use the low osmolality, nonionic CM: the monomeric iopamidol, iohexol, for example, or dimeric, nonionic, blood-isotonic CM preparations (e.g. iotrolan). In these special cases, economic considerations should be less of a priority. From the patient's perspective, however, the lack of taste modifiers in these CM may be a subjective reason for rejecting them.

Angiography of the Gastrointestinal Tract

In addition to endoscopy, isotope examinations and angiography are employed in the investigation of acute or chronic bleeding from the oeso-phagus, stomach, duodenum, small intestine and/or colon. For the detection and localization of a source of bleeding in the GI tract, especially in the small intestine, angiography remains the investigation of choice, if there is active bleeding, with ca. 2 ml of blood per minute passing into the intestinal lumen.

The small intestine is generally visualized by selective angiography of the superior mesenteric artery. In cases of vascular variants, supplementary selective or superselective examinations of the oeliac trunk or its branches sometimes have to be performed. Other indications for angiography of the three major abdominal arteries are clinical questions concerning the vascular anatomy or diagnostically useful pattern of the blood supply of the GI tract or mesenteric tumours. Prior to complex surgery such as pancreatectomy, a surgeon will often wish to be informed about the vascular anatomy. Angio-graphy is used to provide such a "road map".

References

1. Altaras J (1982) Kolon Rektum – Atlas. Urban und Schwarzenberg, München
2. Antes G, Eggemann F (1986) Dünndarmradiologie – Einführung und Atlas. Sprin-ger, Berlin, Heidelberg, New York
3. Cen M, Dihlmann W (1969) Röntgenbefunde am operierten Magen in Abhängigkeit zum postoperativen Intervall. Radiologe 9:187–195
4. Dihlmann W (1976) Die ökonomisch-standardisierte Röntgenuntersuchung des Magens. Dtsch Med Wochenschr 101:900–904
5. Dihlmann W (1980) Die ökonomisch-standardisierte Kontraströntgenuntersuchung des Kolons beim Erwachsenen. Dtsch Med Wochenschr 105:1138–1141
6. Dodds W, Stewart ET, Vlymen WJ (1982) Appropriate contrast media for evaluation of esophageal disruption. Radiology 144:439–441
7. Donner M (1973) Der Schluckvorgang mit saurem Barium. Ein neuartiger Röntgen-test bei Patienten mit Refluxbeschwerden. Radiologe 13:372–376
8. Fernholz HJ, Dihlmann W (1979) Die Bedeutung einer standardisierten Röntgenun-tersuchungstechnik des Magens. Radiologe 190:1–7
9. Frik W (1958) Röntgenuntersuchungen des Magenfeinreliefs. 2. Mitteilung (Untersu-chungstechnik, Kontrastmittelfragen, Diagnostik der chronischen Gastritis, Feinre-lieftechnik bei der Suche nach Antrumkarzinomen). RoFo 88:546–557
10. Frik W, Persigehl M (1990) Ösophagus einschließlich Hypopharynx. In: Radiologi-sche Diagnostik in Klinik und Praxis, 7th edn, vol III/1. Frommhold W, Dihlman W, Stender HS, Thurn P (eds) Thieme, Stuttgart, pp 1–97
11. Holthusen W (1990) Gastrointestinalerkrankungen beim Neugeborenen und beim Kind. In: Radiologische Diagnostik in Klinik und Praxis. 7th edn, vol III/1. Fromm-hold W, Dihlmann W, Stender HS, Thurn P (eds) Thieme, Stuttgart, pp 707–746

12. Hüpscher DN (1988) Radiology of the esophagus. Thieme, Stuttgart
13. Lotz W, Liebenow S (1979) Erweiterte diagnostische Möglichkeiten der röntgenologischen Magenuntersuchung mit verbessertem Kontrastmittel. RoFo 131:157–165
14. Lotz W, Liebenow S (1980) Areae gastricae und varioliforme Erosionen – Qualitätskriterien der röntgenologischen Magenuntersuchung. RoFo 132:491–495
15. Lotz W (1982) Verbesserte röntgenologische Magendiagnostik durch weiterentwikkelte Kontrastmittel und Untersuchungstechnik. Rontgenblatter 35:171–176
16. Miller RE (1978) Die vollständige Colonuntersuchung. Radiologe 15:–410–420
17. Ponette E, Pringot J (1990) Magen. In: Radiologische Diagnostik in Klinik und Praxis. 7th edn, vol III/1. Frommhold W, Dihlmann W, Stender HS, Thurn P (eds) Thieme, Stuttgart, pp 295–476
18. Rubin DL, Caroll BA, Snow HD (1981) The harmful effects of aqueous contrast agents on the gastrointestinal tract: a study of mechanism and means of counteraction. Invest Radiol 16:50–58
19. Schneider V, Maxeiner H (1983) Tödliche Kontrastmittel-Aspiration bei der Röntgenuntersuchung der oberen Speisewege. Munchen Med Wochenschr 125:239–240
20. Sellink JL, Rosenbusch G (1981) Moderne Untersuchungstechnik des Dünndarms oder die 10 Gebote des Enteroklysmas. Radiologe 21:366–376
21. Treichel J (1990) Doppelkontrastuntersuchung des Magens. Untersuchungstechnik und systematische Morphologie der Magenerkrankungen, 2nd edn. Thieme, Stuttgart
22. Treichel J, Oeser H (1975) Die Doppelkontrastmethode: optimale Technik der röntgenologischen Magenuntersuchung. Dtsch Med Wochenschr 100:2226–2229
23. Welin S, Welin G (1980) Die Doppelkontrastuntersuchung des Dickdarms (Erfahrungen mit der Welin-Methode). Thieme, Stuttgart

9.10   Contrast Media in the Gallbladder and Bile Ducts

V. Taenzer

When? Why?

Just a few years ago, an X-ray examination of the biliary system was obligatory for symptoms in the upper abdomen. New imaging and interventional techniques, however, have sharply reduced the importance of cholegraphy. *Oral cholecystography* as a screening method in ill-defined upper abdominal symptoms has been replaced by sonography. Although in gallbladder visualization, the accuracy of the former is roughly as good as that of US, US diagnosis is more reliable. Repeated examinations in cases of negative cholegraphy are obviated. Cholegraphy can be of limited use in individual cases in documenting the size and number of gallstones before and after litholysis.

Intravenous cholangiography/cholecystography has also decreased in importance and is no longer used in jaundice. Endoscopic retrograde cholangiography (ERC), percutaneous transhepatic cholangiography (PTC) and isotope examinations have moved into the forefront here. With normal bilirubin values in serum and normal liver function, good bile duct visualization is achieved by means of intravenous cholangiography, especially in combination with CT of the bile ducts which permits a highly accurate delineation of bile duct abnormalities. The accuracy of roentgenographic bile duct stone recognition, especially where the bile ducts are normal or borderline in width, is not matched by sonography of the bile ducts.

Using intravenous cholegraphy it is possible to make an accurate, reproducible determination of gallstone size. This is very important in modern gallstone treatment since, in the chemolitholysis of gallbladder calculi, progress checks under reproducible conditions are necessary for assessing the success of a given therapy. Even when the new procedure of gallstone lithotripsy is used, an exact determination of size and number of gallstones is necessary preoperatively. In departments where it is technically possible to perform gallstone lithotripsy, the frequency of cholegraphic examinations has once again markedly increasing after an initial period of disuse. Cholegraphy is also indicated in the clarification of uncertain sonographic findings, especially since the competitive procedure of ERC represents a comparatively high risk even in the hands of a practiced endoscopist.

Preconditions

As in all CM delivery, risk factors for hypersensitivity reactions should be conveyed to the radiologist. Communication of the results of US, and possibly CT, are also essential. Furthermore, the request for a cholegraphic examination must state whether there is impaired liver function or jaundice. Special risks such as hyperthyroidism or intolerance of previous administrations of CM have to be ascertained prior to intravenous cholegraphy.

Methods/Procedures

1. *Oral cholegraphy:* A dose of 3–6 g CM is administered perorally 12 h prior to cholegraphy or fractionated 12 and 3 h prior to cholangiography/cholecystography. X-rays are taken with the patient lying and standing, 30 min after administration to assess the contractility of the gallbladder.
2. *Intravenous cholegraphy:* X-ray films are taken 30–120 min after intravenous infusion of 20–30 ml biliary CM, in the early phase in half-hour intervals, in combination with CT of the bile ducts. Otherwise, the examination runs its course as in oral cholegraphy.
3. Where insufficient information is provided by preceding noninvasive investigations in hepatocellular and obstructive jaundice, ERC is used. In cooperation with a physician experienced in endoscopy, the papilla of Vater is probed duodenoscopically and 20–40 ml nonionic uroangiographic CM is administered. ERC permits endoscopic extraction and crushing of bile duct stones; it also allows papillotomy in papillary stenosis and the introduction of internal drainage in bile duct stenoses, whether caused by tumours or not. Because of the possibility of direct thera-

peutic intervention ERC without preceding cholegraphy is used particularly in patients with jaundice.

4. *Percutaneous transhepatic cholangiography:* where ERC cannot be performed, PTC is also used for temporary external biliary drainage, for example in complete stone or tumour obstruction. In PTC, after local anaesthesia and skin puncture, a fine needle is pushed forward with fluoroscopic assistance from the anterolateral abdominal wall to the porta hepatis (so-called Chiba or fine needle). The needle is retracted during simultaneous, slow CM administration. As soon as the needle tip is located in a bile duct, the latter is injected and the entire biliary tract is filled up with nonionic CM.

Complications

1. *Method-induced complications:* In standard noninvasive procedures, there are no special, technique-associated complications. With ERC there is a risk of pancreatitis when there is contrast-visualization of the pancreatic duct. Moreover, the rare risk of clumsy catheterization of the papilla exists, with duodenal perforation and subsequent retroperitoneal abscess formation. PTC is associated with the risk of liver injury, with bleeding and bile peritonitis; in some centres, it is only carried if emergency operation facilities are available.

2. *CM-induced complications:* In intravenous CM administration, both general and organ-specific risks exist, as described elsewhere. The general risk of a hypersensitivity reaction with anaphylactoid shock is severalfold twice as high after injection of biliary CM as it is after the intravenous administration of uroangiographic ionic CM.

Conclusions

US diagnosis and ERC have greatly reduced the importance of standard cholegraphic procedures. A limited range of indications for cholegraphy remains, including chemolitholysis and gallstone lithotripsy and when the sonographic findings are unclear.

9.11 Intravenous Urography

P. Dawson

In spite of the advent of new imaging modalities, the intravenous urogram (IVU) remains the basic technique for the examination of the urinary tract and has the advantage that it is capable of demonstrating the whole of this tract from top to bottom.

Indications

Symptoms and signs referable to the urinary tract.

Contraindications and Precautions

A contraindication to the administration of an intravascular CM is a contraindication to an IVU. The examination is relatively contraindicated in dehydrated patients who may be at risk for CM-associated nephrotoxicity.

Impaired renal function is a relative contraindication as this is believed to be a risk factor for CM-associated renal injury. In severe cases of renal failure the IVU is unlikely to provide much information in any case.

Myeloma and associated conditions are thought to be contraindications because of the alleged danger of precipitation of abnormal proteins and CM molecules in the renal tubules.

Dehydration should be certainly avoided in these conditions if an IVU is performed. The same is true of infants in whom dehydration is dangerous and in whom it may cause distress and crying, movement, etc, which may interfere with the examination.

Choice of Contrast Medium

Any iodinated water-soluble CM may, in principle, be used to obtain an intravenous urogram. A dose of iodine of some 300 mg iodine per kg of patient is generally thought to be suitable.

A few relevant differences between the different kinds of contrast agent should be noted: among the conventional ionic agents, sodium salts tend to produce a lesser osmotic diuresis than meglumine salts and greater urinary contrast concentrations are thereby achieved; the nonionic and low osmolality ionic CM also produce a much lesser osmotic diuresis, resulting in a very significantly increased urinary concentration and pyelographic density than do any of the conventional high osmolality agents.

Dosage

As indicated above, the typical recommended dose is 300 mg iodine per kg for an adult patient. Caution should be exercised in cardiac failure, impaired renal function, in the elderly and in paediatric patients. Many radiologists prefer to use nonionic agents in all these cases.

It is difficult to pontificate about paediatric doses but a similar dosage regimen on a weight basis as for adults may be used. In general, doses in any situation must always be tailored to the patient's clinical state.

Patient Preparation

1. Nil by mouth for 4–6 h prior to the examination. The aim is to achieve an empty stomach in case of an adverse reaction rather than to dehydrate the patient.
2. Bowel preparation is performed by some departments. It entails a risk of dehydration and, some would argue, that with the availability of simple tomography it is not nearly so necessary as in the past.
3. If the patient is thought to be at particular risk from an adverse reaction to the CM but the examination must, nevertheless, proceed, the use of a nonionic agent, possibly with corticosteroid or antihistamine prophylaxis should be considered (See Sects. 5.5, 5.6).

Plain Films

1. A supine full-length anteroposterior (AP) film of the abdomen should be obtained. The lower border of the film should be at the level of the symphysis pubis with the beam centered at iliac crest level.
2. Supine AP films of the renal areas in inspiration and expiration may be taken as appropriate in order to determine whether any plain film calcifications are likely to lie within the kidneys.

An opacity apparently in, or overlying, the kidneys may be further elucidated by:
a) oblique views,
b) plain tomography through the kidneys or
c) inspiration and expiration views of the renal areas.

Contrast Administration

An antecubital vein is chosen for contrast adminstration and, using a 19G needle usually in adults but a smaller needle in children, a rapid bolus injection of the CM (less than 1 min) is given. Care should be taken not to extravasate the CM.

Film Sequences

Immediate Nephrogram. Immediately at the end of the injection an AP film is taken of the renal areas and will demonstrate the nephrogram, which consists principally of CM filtered into the proximal tubules of the kidney.

Five-Minute Film. An AP film is taken of the renal areas again after about 5 min. At this point in the normal kidney excretion should be obvious in the pelvicaliceal system. Abdominal compression is usually now applied in order to produce pelvicaliceal system distension. Compression may, however, be contraindicated in: (a) recent abdominal or renal trauma, (b) abdominal mass, (c) recent abdominal surgery, or (d) when the 5-min film has demonstrated a dilated collecting system.

Ten-Minute Film. An AP film of the renal areas may again be taken to demonstrate the renal collecting system in a fully distended state.

Release Film. A supine AP abdominal film is repeated and should demonstrate the whole urinary tract with some filling of the bladder at some 20 min or so after the CM injection.

Other. Specific bladder views may be obtained before and after micturition and residual volumes assessed.

Additional Films

Like all radiological examinations, the IVU must be tailored to the patient and modifications to the standard technique must be introduced as necessary as the examination evolves. Thus the following may be considered in some patients:
1. Oblique views of the kidneys or bladder
2. Tomography
3. The visualisation of the ureters may be better with the patient prone, particularly if there is a pelvi-uteric junction (PUJ) obstruction.
4. If a PUJ obstruction is suspected an intravenous injection of a loop diuretic such as frusemide mide may be given in order to precipitate such an obstruction.
5. Delayed films may be taken in cases of an obstructive nephropathy in order to try to see some CM excretion and to delineate the level of the obstruction.

Special Cases

1. *Patients with significant renal impairment,* in particular, must never be dehydrated. Preliminary tomography may be necessary to determine optimal tomography levels for the visualization of the kidneys. A higher dose than usual of CM should be given though, the possibility that it will further impair on renal function must be borne in mind. Tomography during the early nephrographic phase should be performed. Delayed films are usually necessary.
2. *In hypertensive patients* some radiologists like to perform very rapid intravenous bolus injection followed by rapid sequence films of the renal

areas to detect a discrepancy in the timing of the appearance of the pyelogram which might indicate a renal artery stenosis. It should be noted, however, that this technique is far from reliable in detecting a renal artery stenosis.

3. A fizzy drink may be given to *infants* to produce a dilated, gas-filled stomach to act as a window through which the kidneys may be seen. The right posterior oblique (RPO) position may be useful in visualization of the right kidney. Tomography may be necessary, though this increases the radiation dose.

Abdominal compression is usually avoided in very young children.

Excretion of CM may be delayed in the first month of life and optimum visualization of the urinary tract occurs at up to 3 h, which clearly dictates a modification of the usual technique.

Cystography

A cystogram is obtained routinely in an IVU if the kidneys are functioning. It should be noted that with the low osmolality agents the osmotic diuresis is reduced and filling of the bladder delayed. This may lengthen the examination. Oblique views of the bladder, tomography, and even attempts at double-contrast cystography by the use of a lead-gloved hand bladder compression during fluoroscopy have all been used to seek bladder pathology. However, it should be understood that this is usually inadequate to completely exclude bladder pathology and if there is a serious suspicion, cystoscopy must be performed.

9.12 Urethrography and Micturating Cystography, Cavernosography, and Seminal Vesiculography and Vasography

D. Rickards

Urethrography and Micturating Cystography

Introduction

Urethrography and micturating cystography will be considered together as they are inextricably entwined. Any suspected lower tract pathology or vesicoureteric reflux form the indications for these studies. Since the first urethrogram performed by Cunningham in 1910 [1], many CM have been used, including barium and Lipiodol. What is needed, according to Kaufman and Russell [2], is an agent that is:

a) of adequate radiopacity,
b) of adequate viscosity,
c) miscible with urine and water,
d) safe in the vascular circulation and
e) sterile.

Once oily CM had been deemed dangerous because of pulmonary oil emboli [1], manufacturers tried to fulfil the above criteria by producing specialized agents for urethrography, e.g. Umbradil-Viscous (Astra) and Thixokon (Mallinckrodt). Both these agents were viscous enough to dilate the urethra and were used up until 1970, when they were withdrawn because of potentially inadequate sterility and replaced by ionic CM, e.g. Conray 280 (May and Baker) and Urografin 310M (Schering). To increase the viscosity of these agents, they can be mixed with sterile KY jelly, gum acacia or Lubafax (Burroughs Wellcome). Lubafax is the agent of choice, but such thickening agents are rarely needed and are best avoided.

Micturating cystography requires a CM that has volume up to 500 ml (and very often more is needed) is sterile and of adequate density.

In the UK, the only agent that fulfils these criteria is Urografin 150 (Schering AG) which is supplied in 250-ml and 500-ml bottles.

Technique

Full assessment of the urethra involves both an ascending and descending urethrogram. The patient should be questioned about his present drug regimen, allergies and any previous contrast examination. No preparation is required unless the patient is very nervous or has a history of an autonomic disorder, in which circumstances it is advisable to administer 0.6 mg atropine prior to the procedure.

Ascending Urethrography. There are many commercially available penile clamps that are used to instil CM into the external meatus, e.g. Cunningham, Knutsen. Individual choice determines which one is suitable. The use of a Foley catheter, the balloon of which is partially inflated in the navicular fossa of the anterior urethra to provide a water-tight seal, is to be avoided because
a) it is more than likely that the balloon will be blown up in the anterior urethra and not the navicular fossa,
b) it is painful and
c) the balloon causes urethral trauma.

Before the study, the patient should try and empty his bladder, preferably combined with uroflowmetry. Once in place, contrast is instilled slowly under fluoroscopic control with the patient in the supine oblique position and relevant films of the anterior urethra exposed. Adequate distension of

the anterior urethra can be obtained without thickening agents by injecting CM more rapidly. In ascending urethrography, resistance to retrograde injection will be afforded by the distal sphincter or constricting anterior urethral pathology, e.g. stricture. Overdistension should be avoided because of pain and the possibility of intravasation. Ideally, CM should pass proximal to the distal sphincter to outline the posterior urethra. Contrast may not pass proximally into the bladder because
a) of obstructing anterior urethral pathology,
b) of spasm of the distal sphincter mechanism,
c) obstructing posterior urethral pathology or
d) bladder neck spasm or stenosis.

If there is no suprapubic catheter in situ through which the bladder can be filled, the examination is ended. Distal sphincter spasm may pass with time, but the administration of muscle relaxants is worthless.

Descending Micturating Cystourethrography. Contrast has to be instilled into the bladder either by
a) retrograde filling via the penile clamp in males,
b) via a suprapubic catheter or
c) via a urethral catheter.

Suprapubic and urethral catheters have the advantage of being able to drain the bladder before filling, thus accurately assessing the amount of residual urine and avoiding dilution of any contrast instilled into the bladder that would diminish anatomical detail. In order for the patient to initiate micturition, the bladder has to be adequately filled and what volume is required is dependent upon the patient's urodynamic status. The normal adult bladder is capable of containing 500 ml without difficulty, but the patient that has been on suprapubic catheter drainage for more than 7 days or has detrusor instability is likely to tolerate only a much lower volume. During filling, the bladder anatomy is noted on fluoroscopy and relevant films exposed. When a male feels full, but not overfull (such a situation is likely to inhibit micturition), he voids either supine (male) or erect in the prone oblique position and spot films of the posterior urethra are exposed. Females void into a specially designed funnel held between their upper thighs while standing and films are exposed in the anteroposterior position. Whilst under direct fluoroscopy, the patient is asked to voluntarily stop micturition at any stage before complete bladder emptying. In males and under normal circumstances, the distal sphincter should immediately shut and the small amount of CM within the posterior urethra will be milked back into the bladder through the bladder neck. In addition, the anterior urethra should empty completely. Any CM left in any part of the urethra either during the "stop test" or at the end of micturition is abnormal. In females, the distal sphincter should close, but emptying of the urethra with milk back into the bladder is the exception rather than the rule. The female bladder neck is often incompetent in nulliparous young females and it is not a structure that is essential to urinary continence.

Combined anterior and descending micturating urethrography provides the following information:
1. Anatomy of the urethra
2. Bladder capacity
3. Bladder anatomy
4. Presence or abscence of vesicoureteric reflux
5. Competence of the bladder neck
6. Competence of the distal sphincter
7. Presence or absence of intraprostatic reflux
8. Residual urine volume.

Complications

Pain. Adequate distension of the anterior urethra is associated with pain which can be eliminated by the administration of lignocaine jelly prior to the study. However, lignocaine jelly is very viscous and when injected into the urethra causes a lot of distension of it and, consequently, pain. Lignocaine jelly also reduces the quality of the radiographs by causing filling defects in the urethra.

Haemorrhage. In some patients, especially those with urethral pathology, distension causes small mucosal capillary tears and subsequent haemorrhage and does not detract from the quality of the study.

Intravasation. Intravasation is due either to:
a) the intraurethral part of the delivery system used impinging upon the distal anterior urethral mucosa – this is faulty technique – or
b) overdistension in the presence of urethral pathology.

In either event, the procedure must be terminated and the patient given prophylactic antibiotics. Intravasation is associated with heavy postprocedural haemorrhage which is usually self-limiting.

Reactions to Contrast Media. Reactions to CM are less likely to occur than with intravenous contrast administrations and more likely if intravasation occurs. Ionic CM are usually used for luminal studies because of cost considerations. Should the patient have any allergic history, nonionic agents should be considered, but to fill the bladder with 500 ml of nonionic contrast is expensive. In the author's clinical practice, nonionic CM have not been used for any urethral study.

Infection. Any instrumentation of the lower urinary tract is liable to be complicated by infection, especially if there is a urodynamic abnormality, e.g. incomplete bladder emptying. Antibiotics should be considered in those patients who leave large bladder residuals, are known to have an urinary tract infection and in whom bleeding occurs as a result of the study.

Cavernosography

Cavernosography involves the direct administration of CM directly into the corpora cavernosa. The indications are: impotence, painful or deviant erection, or, following suspected penile fracture.

Different CM requirements are to be met, depending upon the indication for the study which must be considered as an intravascular procedure. For anatomical depiction of the corpora (indications 1 and 2), the CM needs to be of adequate radioopacity sterile, and nontoxic in the subcutaneous tissues.

These requirements are met by a nonionic medium that contains between 250–300 mg% iodine. In our practice, Omnipaque 300 is used.

In the investigation of impotence, cavernosography is performed as part of a penile pressure study to assess the response of erectile tissue to muscle relaxants, e.g. papaverine, and perfusion of CM at known rates. CM requirements are: adequate radiopacity, viscosity and volume and that it is sterile and nontoxic in the subcutaneous space.

Up to 500 ml may be used, but in 90% of studies 200 ml is sufficient. The CM is injected via a pressure pump at a rate between 15 and 20 ml/min and so cannot be too viscous. In our practice, the ideal medium is Omnipaque 300 (Nycomed) or Niopam 300 (Bracco) diluted 50:50 with normal saline.

Technique

Cavernosography. A single 21-gauge butterfly needle is inserted into either corpus as distally as possible, preferably just proximal to the glans penis. Under fluoroscopic control, CM is slowly injected and both copora are opacified. Up to 40 ml CM will be needed to opacify both corpora, which freely intercommunicate. Spot films in the relevant degree of obliquity are exposed.

The needle is withdrawn and the site of puncture compressed until no bleeding can be identified. The following information can be gained: anatomy of the corpora and normal venous drainage.

Pharmacocavernometrography. Pharmacocavernometrography involves both corpora being punctured with 21-gauge butterfly needles as distally in the corpora as possible. Through one needle, continuous pressure measurements are recorded by connecting it to a pressure transducer. Through the other, muscle relaxants and CM are injected. Whilst CM is being injected, the patient should be turned supine oblique so that the whole length of the corpora can be seen fluoroscopically and the draining veins at the base of the corpora identified. Spot films of the relevant anatomy are exposed. The information gained is: corporal dynamics, corporal anatomy and anatomy of the draining veins.

Complications

Extravasation. Contrast which is injected into the pericorporal tissues is associated with instant localized pain and the needle must be repositioned. Extravasation is easily identified on fluoroscopy as the CM will not flow away from the tip of the needle on injection.

Contrast Reactions. A full allergy history must be taken. However, the use of ionic CM should be avoided as they are more toxic in the extravascular space.

Priapism. Priapism is a complication of the muscle relaxants given to achieve erection rather than the CM used.

Corporal Rupture. This is a complication of poor technique. If the corpora are overdistended by too rapid a rate of injection, rupture is possible and serious because it is itself a cause of impotence.

Infection. Infection is rare as long as aseptic measures are taken.

Seminal Vesiculography and Vasography

Seminal vesiculography and vasography are part of the investigation of obstructive infertility and involve the direct administration of CM into the vas deferens and/or seminal vesicles. Transrectal US has partly replaced these procedures, but where that fails to identify the level of obstruction, contrast studies are indicated. The CM should be of adequate radioopacity, nonirritant to the mucosa of the vas deferens, of low viscosity and sterile. Many agents fulfil these criteria. In our practice, Omnipaque 240 (Nycomed) is used.

Technique

Vasography is usually performed in theatre immediately prior to corrective surgery to any obstructing lesion that may be identified. The vas is surgically exposed in the scrotum and cannulated. CM is injected under image intensification control until either there is flow of CM seen into the posterior urethra, which excludes an obstructing lesion, or there is hold-up of CM despite adequate injection pressure, which indicates the level of an obstructing lesion.

Seminal vesiculography aims to identify the patency of the seminal vesicle ducts. This can be done by (a) cannulating the ejaculatory ducts at urethroscopy – this will also provide opacification of the vas deferens – or (b) puncturing the seminal vesicles via a perineal approach under transrectal US control. This is likely to give information about the seminal vesicle and ejaculatory ducts only.

In either approach, sufficient contrast is injected until the relevant anatomy has been detailed and spot films exposed.

Complications

Infection. As with any invasive procedure, infection is a possible complication but this is rare as a sterile procedure is easily attained.

Haemospermia. Though alarming of the patient, this is an important finding as it indicates patency of the ejaculatory ducts.

Pain. Overdistension of the seminal vesicles causes perineal pain.

References

1. Cunningham JR (1990) The diagnosis of stricture of the urethra by the roentgen rays. Trans Amer Assoc Genitourinary Surgeons 5: 369
2. Kaufmann JJ, Russell M (1959) Cystourethrography: clinical experience with newer contrast agents. Am J Roentgenol 75:884

9.13 The Kidneys and Adrenal Glands

G. P. Krestin

Computed Tomography of the Kidneys and Adrenal Glands

Why?

Shortly after the introduction of CT as a noninvasive imaging technique, its importance for the routine diagnosis of pathological changes in the retroperitoneum became clear. Already by 1980, a cost reduction of more than 30% vis-à-vis 1973 could be reached through the use of CT for the clarification of renal masses. As regards this question, CT has to compete today effectively only with US, whereas standard X-ray procedures are primarily employed for the assessment of the urinary tract.

For detecting adrenal mass lesions, CT clearly represents the technique of first choice. Its outstanding importance has been in no way diminished in recent years by the use of MRI. In the renal region, MRI can at best be used as a supplementary technique, especially in patients who demonstrate a known intolerance to iodinated CM. In adrenal gland imaging, a more-reliable differentiation of pathological processes is possible with MRI, but CT still remains the recommended method of detection due to its better spatial resolution.

One advantage of CT over US consists in the possibility of using CM. Not only are organ blood flow and pathological changes made visible in this way, but kidney excretion can also be visualized. Dynamic sequences may permit a semi-quantitative estimation of renal function.

When?

Today, CT is usually used as a supplementary technique to US. Here it is often a question of confirming or characterizing an already detected pathological lesion or of confirming or excluding suspected change.

CT is rarely used for clarifying the nature of inflammatory renal disorders; if at all, it is performed in cases of abscesses or xanthogranulomatous pyelonephritis. Cysts are usually identified sonographically; if uncertainties remain, CT can provide further information and better differentiate between "simple" and "complicated" cysts. All uncharacterized cysts and cystic and solid masses can be identified using CT. In some cases, this yields an aetiological classification (e.g. angiomyolipoma) and after CM administration usually a precise localization and determination of the extent of the pathological change. For the preoperative staging of renal cell carcinoma, CT is the technique of choice.

In the adrenal gland region, it is a question of recording pathological changes: CT is here the best "screening" procedure for detecting or excluding adrenal gland metastases as well as benign adrenal gland enlargements (hyperplasia, adenoma). When CM is administered it is possible to differentiate between well-developed and less well-developed vascular lesions. The indications for CM administration in CT examination of the renal and adrenal gland region have been summarized in Table 9.13.1.

How?

In order for an investigation to provide useful diagnostic information the kidney and adrenal gland region should be imaged both before and after CM administration. A complete set of 8- to 10-mm-thick, contiguous slices should be made for precontrast inspection. Only when searching for small calcifications is thin-slice tomography (2- to 5-mm slices) required before CM is administered.

For the diagnosis of perirenal and pararenal masses, investigating more extensive inflammation, or for excluding the possibility of a local residuum after tumour nephrectomy, peroral contrast enhancement of the upper gas-

Table 9.13.1. Use of CM in CT diagnosis in the kidneys and adrenal glands

CM use	Indications
Kidneys	
Not necessary	Detection of stones, angiomyolipoma, hydronephrosis, large cysts
Helpful	Tumour detection, tumour differentiation
Diagnostic	Abscesses, assessment of function, infarct
Adrenal glands	
Not necessary	Hyperplasia, exclusion of tumour
Helpful	For better differentiation and detection of the tumour's composition (necroses, cystic parts)
Diagnostic	Differentiation of hypervascularized lesions (pheochromocytomas, carcinomas)

trointestinal tract is also required. For this, solutions such as 500–800 ml of 4% Gastrografin are used.

CT Angiography. One administers typically 60–100 ml CM at a flow of 8–10 ml/s. Films of the kidneys are then taken in rapid succession 20–25 s after the introduction of the CM bolus. Slices should be 5–8 mm thick. The technique is well suited for visualizing the cortico-medullary junction; this is best accomplished about 20–100 s after CM administration. Since the whole kidney cannot be visualized in this way, one should set the focus on the region of interest beforehand.

There are only a few indications for renal CT angiography. Renal perfusion and a possible renal infarct can be registered earlier and more effectively in this way. Moreover, more information can be gained in the diagnosis of kidney transplant dysfunction. CT angiography is unsuitable for the detection or differentiation of adrenal gland pathology.

Contrast-Enhanced Images. Adequate visualization of the kidneys and adrenal glands is typically reached 5–10 min after rapid administration of 100 ml CM. The kidneys can be examined with 8- to 10-mm contiguous slices and the adrenal glands with 5-mm slices. In the case of a pathological finding, especially if its diameter is under 1.5 cm, thin-slice images (2- to 4-mm slices) should be carried out in order to record precisely the size of the lesion. In this way, distortions in the measurement due to partial volume effects can usually be avoided. If the patients are incapable of cooperating very much and, due to variable inspiration the changes to be visualized can only be recorded poorly or not at all, it is advisable to take 5-mm slices, with 3-mm table shifts. Here it has to be taken into account that CT is often the last diagnostic examination before surgery and it should be conducted as carefully as possible.

Complications

Complications in renal CT can be caused by systemic effects of the CM itself (described elsewhere in this book), by the route and rate of CM administration and by the possibly diseased condition of the organ of interest (renal functional disorder).

Slight side effects from CM administration such as feeling sick, hot or nauseous, frequently occur at high administration rates. For this reason, it is not uncommon after bolus administration to have to interrupt the examination for a short period, ultimately leading to a suboptimal examination. Bolus administration of CM should, therefore, not always be used, but only.

The nephrotoxic effect of iodinated CM is greater in patients with previously impaired renal function (e.g. chronic glomerulonephritis, diabetic nephropathy). Pre-existing dehydration increases risk of nephrotoxicity. Another form of nephrotoxicity is caused by pathological protein (Tamm-Horsfall mucoprotein and Bence Jones protein) precipitates and uric acid precipitates. The incidence of serious renal functional disorder following intravenous CM administration can be markedly reduced by sufficient hydration of the patients prior to testing. Hence, a longer fast before renal CT examination should be avoided in all patients.

Conclusion

The use of CM plays an essential role in renal and adrenal gland CT imaging. Aside from the distinction between nonvascular, poorly vascular, and highly vascular lesions, the possibility of a semi-quantitative assessment of renal function also exists. Both bolus injection and infusion produce powerful enhancement of the properly functioning renal parenchyma, and there are only a few clinical indications for CT angiography and it is often more poorly tolerated by patients. Thus, rapid CM infusion is sufficient for most purposes.

Renal and Adrenal Gland Angiograms

Why?

Renal vessels can be visualized directly following intraarterial contrast injection or, indirectly, by intravenous CM administration (indirect intravenous digital subtraction angiography). The renal veins can be enhanced indirectly after intraarterial CM injection or, in a retrograde manner, by means of direct intravenous CM injection. For the visualization of adrenal gland arteries, selective arterial CM injection is required.

All so-called noninvasive procedures allow only indirect assessment of vascular anatomy and possible intraluminal lesions. Even if the results of

CT, "real-time" US or MRI sometimes suggest a lesion, ultimately vascular stenosis can only be reliably detected or excluded on the basis of angiography. Doppler US is the only noninvasive technique yielding some information about haemodynamics. However, possible multiple feeders, pathological vascular structures or damage to the intima following trauma can be delineated only on an angiogram.

When?

Angiograms are by nature invasive examinations and thus represent considerable stress on patients and angiography is only justified given a clear indication, i.e. if there is a high probability of influencing therapy as a result. Absolute indications for angiography are the suspicion of renal artery stenosis and the clarification of possible renal vessel injury. The diagnosis of renal and adrenal gland tumours is today at best only an occasional indication for angiography, which is indicated principally for pre-operative visualization of vascularity. Renal and adrenal gland phlebography is carried out only in exceptional cases.

How?

For most questions posed today, digital subtraction angiography (DSA) has replaced standard (cut-film) angiography. The DSA technique also has the advantage of indirect vascular visualization following intravenous CM administration. The indications for intravenous DSA of the renal arteries have to be clearly distinguished from those requiring intraarterial DSA.

Intravenous DSA of the Renal Arteries. The elucidation of renovascular hypertension, the suspicion of renal artery embolism, follow-up examinations after an operation or percutaneous angioplasty and the securing of a diagnosis in a solitary kidney are indications for IV CM visualization.

The examination is carried out after introducing a central venous high-pressure catheter via the basilic vein with intestinal hypotonia (40 mg Buscopan i.v.) and, if at all possible, using ECG triggering. On average, two to three series of films are taken sagittally as well as at a 20° left oblique or a 30°–45° right oblique. Per series, 35–40 ml of a 60% CM are administered with a flow rate of 20 ml/s. With this technique, the examination is diagnostic in 95% of cases (accuracy, 90%; sensitivity, 86%; specificity, 92%).

Intra-arterial DSA of the Renal Arteries. Angiography with intraarterial CM administration is indicated in the following cases: if intravenous DSA has not provided a diagnosis or is unclear, during percutaneous angioplasty, for kidney transplant study (rejection or stenosis), preoperatively for the clarification of vascularity or of venous involvement, or in the kidney donor, in cases of suspected renal vein thrombosis and in suspected traumatic vascular lesions.

In the examination of the renal arteries a pigtail catheter is first introduced as a rule via the femoral artery. This permits a survey study of the abdominal aorta with the administration of 25 ml of a 60% CM (flow rate 15–20 ml/min). For selective angiography, a special catheter (renal, cobra or side-winder catheter) is substituted. One or more series are taken sagittally or obliquely after administering 20 ml CM (at a flow rate of 8 ml/s) per series.

Cut-Film Angiography of the Renal Arteries. Cut-film angiography is still indicated for noncompliant patients, for extremely obese patients and before transluminal angioplasty in order to determine the exact diameter of the vessel.

The same examination technique is used as in intra-arterial DSA but about 35–40 ml CM are administered per series. Sharpness of detail can be increased by using magnification techniques. The intraarterial administration of vasodilators or vasoconstrictors (pharmacoangiography) may facilitate tumour diagnosis.

Renal Phlebography. Renal phlebography is only used in exceptional cases. It can be combined with venous blood sampling. It is, however no longer indicated for the diagnosis of tumour thrombosis. DSA is used in the renal phlebographic examination after catheterization of the femoral vein.

Adrenal Gland Angiography. The visualization of adrenal gland vessels is preoperatively indicated in the case of a proven space-occupying mass. Today, this examination is predominantly carried out with intraarterial DSA technique and cut-film angiography is only used on noncompliant or extremely obese patients. Flush abdominal aortography is first performed in order to determine the vascularity of large adrenal or extra-adrenal tumours. Selective angiography is performed by catheterization of the renal vessels or by selective catheterization of the adrenal gland arteries. Pinpoint diagnosis can be obtained by means of magnification techniques. 5–10 ml CM are manually administered superselectively.

Adrenal Gland Phlebography. Selective adrenal gland phlebography is performed by catheterization of the veins with special catheters. Retrograde visualization of the entire adrenal gland can be achieved by manual CM injection. The phlebography of adrenal gland veins is usually only carried out today in selective venous blood sampling in hormonal overproduction.

Complications

Alongside the general complications already described arising from the actual administration of CM (see renal and adrenal gland CT), arteriography is subject to a variety of complications. Local complications at the site of the puncture frequently occur when higher-caliber catheters are used or catheters are frequently changed. In the selective catheterization of renal vessels, intimal dissection or thromboembolism, though rare, may occur. This can induce an acute increase in blood pressure. In selective renal angiography, vasoconstriction and vasospasm are observed frequently, above all in the segmental arteries, as compared to other vessels. They usually resolve spontaneously or can be abolished by medication. There is a naturally higher frequency of complications in the course of renal artery interventions.

In adrenal gland angiography, if a pheochromocytoma is present, hypertensive crises can be triggered. Thus, given a known or suspected pheochromocytoma, long-term prophylaxis with alpha (or alpha and beta) receptor blockers should be undertaken prior to planned angiography. In selective adrenal gland phlebography, the administration of CM at high pressure can easily lead to extravasation, haematoma or infarct.

Conclusions

The main indication for renal angiography today is the elucidation of renovascular hypertension. In contrast, diagnostic angiography for the diagnosis of renal masses is only rarely justified, whereas adrenal gland angiography has practically been abandoned. With careful execution and selection of procedure, and the sparing use of CM, even this invasive imaging technique is associated only rarely with complications.

9.14 Contrast Media in Gynaecology

H. J. Maurer and *J. G. Heep*

Hysterosalpingography

Why?

The indications for hysterosalpingography (HSG) have only been reduced in part by US, which avoids the use of ionizing rays. The extent to which MRI will also further limit the use of HSG depends upon its spatial resolution. US can generally demonstrate the uterus and ovaries precisely enough, but its spatial resolving power is not (yet) sufficient to image the fallopian tubes. Here, however, the incorporation of US CM into US practice could lead to an increase in the range of its indications.
1. Today, HSG is primarily used to examine variants and malformations of the internal female genitalia, especially with regard to tubal patency and

spill and possible obstruction; the form and extent of pathological chan-ges in the ovarian fimbria can also be better demonstrated with HSG than US.

2. HSG is also indicated for examining the tubes before and after their ligation or before and after reconstruction operations.
3. Some centres perform HSG prior to intracavitary radiotherapy in cases of uterine body or cervical carcinoma in order to gain a precise image of the location and extent of the carcinoma. This procedure, however, is largely being replaced by US and hysteroscopy.

When?

Since HSG is an invasive technique using ionizing radiation, it should follow all non-invasive examination procedures; for example, in fertility tests, it should only be used after the endocrinological and andrological tests have been completed. The only exception is if a malformation or pathological change, such as sactosalpinx, has already been detected clinically or by US and requires further clarification. HSG should be performed, following clinical and US exams, if possible, in the first 14 days following menstrua-tion.

How?

The instrumentation used for performing HSG is well known. Increasing-ly, use is being made of the suction technique, which does not injure the portio cervicalis. Only in very rare cases does the cervical canal have to be dilated. Whether HSG should be performed (a) under local anaesthesia or (b) while holding the cervical os depends upon the examiner or the ana-tomical situation. General anaesthesia has its own risks and is only neces-sary in atypical situations in which the patient is under emotional stress or frightened. A genital infection has to be excluded or cleared up prior to HSG.

HSG has to be performed under locally sterile conditions in order to prevent the introduction of organisms into the cervix and corpus uteri. The nonionic, iodinated CM (20 ml, 300 mg I/ml) is administered under fluoro-scopic control. The required images should be in medium format (100 mm) with an image intensifier in order to use the smallest possible dose of radiation, ca. 20% of a standard image.

Complications

Technique-Related Complications. As the instrument is inserted, injuries to the cervical wall, though very rare, or perforations of it, though even rarer, can occur. This may happen if the cervical wall has been softened by inflammation or (very rarely) by tumour.

During or after HSG, bleeding can occur as a result of injury to a blood vessel of the ostium uteri, as in the case of a small, submucosal, invisible haemangioma, or injury to the cervical mucous membrane. This can also occur if a (previously unknown) coagulopathy exists. Such bleeding can usually be stopped locally.

X-Ray Contrast Media-Related Complications. Even in a properly performed HSG, a small amount of the X-ray CM can be absorbed by the mucous membrane. In spite of fluoroscopic monitoring, occasionally too much CM is injected, especially in cases of a completely closed cervical canal or fallopian tubes closed on one or both sides. Even with normal injection pressure, CM may penetrate the uterine wall and intravasat to veins and/or lymphatic vessels.

In patent tubes, a greater or lesser amount of the X-ray CM makes its way into the abdominal cavity. Here it is quickly absorbed. Peritoneal irritation and general side effects caused by systemic X-ray CM effects after absorption are rare. Nonionic, low-osmolar X-ray CM and the isotonic X-ray CM iotrolan have proven to be especially well tolerated.

Lymphography of the Groin, Pelvic and Paravertebral Area

Why?

Imaging of the lymphatic vessels and nodes primarily serves for the detection of metastases. The sensitive imaging methods of US, CT and MRI have largely reduced the need for lymphography, especially since the specificity of the last is insufficient to fulfil all expectations. Moreover, the further development of radio- and chemotherapy has now made the precision formerly required in lymph-node assessment superfluous.

When?

If in suspected lymphnode metastases the imaging procedures just cited have not provided adequate information, lymphography can aid diagnosis by detecting changes characteristic of metastases in normal-sized lymphnodes themselves or in lymphatic vessels in the pelvic or paravertebral area.

How?

See the section on lymphography.

Complications?

See the section on lymphography.

Lymphography of the Breast

Why?

Despite many efforts, a satisfactory technique for the lymphography of the breast has not yet been successfully developed, especially one that would permit the axillary, supraclavicular and parasternal lymphnodes to be adequately demonstrated too.

When?

If at all, lymphography of the breast should be performed at the end of the diagnostic process, in order to aid in treatment decisions.

Phlebography

Why?

In signs of swelling of one or both of the lower extremities, phlebography can help to make the diagnosis: thrombosis of the external and/or common iliac veins and its cranial spread (inferior vena cava); or, compression caused by tumour or lymph nodes.

The imaging of the uterine plexus and the deep pelvic veins to exclude postpartum thrombosis without operation is not possible by means of persymphyseal or pertrochanteric injection or through peruterine CM injection in the two cornua corpus uteri. This question may be resolved using US or by MRI if their spatial resolving power proves sufficient.

When?

Phlebography of the pelvic veins is indicated if clinical examination, Doppler US, CT and/or MRI have not yielded an unequivocal explanation of the cause of swelling of one or both of the lower extremities and lymphoedema has been excluded. The technique of phlebography, its complications and their treatment are discussed in the section on phlebography (Sect. 9.4).

Arteriography of the Internal Genitalia

Why?

Though many efforts have been made to expand diagnostic accuracy with the help of arteriography, the procedure has failed to become established. The arteriographic findings were not characteristic enough to contribute to definitive diagnosis. Only in cases of hydatid mole/choriocarcinoma is it possible, on the basis of an angiographic roadmap to make the staging classification that is crucial for treatment decisions.

When?

Arteriography of the internal genitalia is not used until all other diagnostic imaging procedures have been tried, unless there are special reasons in individual cases requiring a change in this sequence (US → CT/MRI → arteriography).

How?

Examination is always carried out using the Seldinger technique. A pigtail catheter is used for the aortography, whereas an appropriately preformed catheter is employed for selective examinations (see also Sect. 9.3, 9.7).

Arteriography of the Breast

Why?

Basically, the same holds for the arteriography of the breast as for the internal genitalia. The findings are largely nonspecific and are, thus, seldom of decisive significance.

When?

Arteriography of the mammary vessels is generally employed as the last of the imaging procedures (US → mammography → MRI → arteriography).

How?

Arteriography is performed transfemorally using the Seldinger technique with an appropriately preformed catheter is inserted into the internal thoracic (mammary) artery.

Complications and their treatment are discussed in the chapter on arteriography. (See Sect. 9.3.)

9.15 Arthrography

V. Papassotiriou

Why?

Arthrography continues to be a valuable examination technique in the imaging of joint disorders in spite of the introduction and spread of endoscopy and modern imaging techniques such as US, CT and MRI. It provides comprehensive data on the condition of the menisci and discs, the thickness of, and changes in, articular cartilage, lesions of the ligamentous apparatus and the size, form, contents and parietal contours of the capsules and their bursae and recessus.

As a virtually low-risk technique, arthrography is associated with no sequelae and thus can usually be performed on outpatients. It can be used on children and elderly patients without reservation. Arthrography is a very easy technique to perform and requires no special equipment. It can be carried out in any practice possessing standard equipment. For this reason, it is less costly than CT or MRI.

A very important advantage of the technique is its great diagnostic power and accuracy. In the hands of experienced users and with careful technique, arthrography may attain a diagnostic accuracy of 90%–95% [1, 9].

The use of standard tomography and CT after the administration of X-ray CM, or X-ray CM and air or gas (oxygen, carbon dioxide) markedly extends the range of possibilities provided by the technique to address specific diagnostic questions.

When?

Arthrography should always be preceded by a careful clinical examination of the joint and its function. The clinical examination provides the indispensable basis for deciding which special diagnostic procedures are subsequently indicated.

It is also absolutely necessary first to obtain conventional films of the joints. This may reveal the following causes of clinical symptoms: osseous lesions following trauma, inflammation of bone and joint, degenerative processes, aseptic necroses, loose radiopaque intra-articular bodies, calcification of the menisci and articular cartilage, and tumours.

Accordingly, arthrography should be employed largely to clarify the suspected clinical diagnosis, i.e. to confirm or exclude it and to secure support for further therapeutic measures.

The indications for arthrography vary somewhat for different joints:

Arthrography of the knee joint is performed most frequently. Data on its frequency, however, vary considerably. According to Hall [4], it accounts

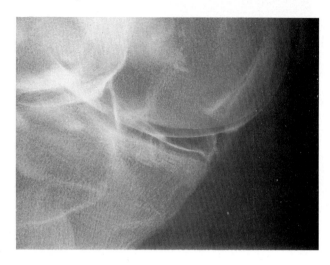

Fig. 9.15.1. Positive single-contrast arthrography of the knee joint (10 ml Iotrolan 300) in a 25-year-old patient after a sports accident. Diagnosis: longitudinal rupture of the medial meniscus near the capsule

for 55% of all arthrographic examinations, according to Dalinka [2] and my own statistics, 80%–90%.

The indications for knee-joint arthrography are: acute trauma; sport- and work-related accidents with articular distortion (Fig. 9.15.1); unexplained recurring haematomas with and without trauma; chronic, nonspecific joint symptoms; persisting symptoms following endoscopic intervention or arthrotomy; articular "locking" due to meniscal lesions or loose bodies in the joint, mostly in osteochondritis dissecans; nonspecific swelling in the posterior articular space and along the calf muscles; and articular instability and meniscal injuries in athletes and patients subject to occupationally related strains (e.g. floor tilers, gardeners, etc.). Another important area in which arthrography of the knee joint is indicated arises when expert opinion is needed, especially in cases of doubt involving work-related accidents or previous interventions.

The following are held to be the most important indications for *arthrography of the shoulder:* impact trauma and arm distortion with delayed mobilisation and shoulder symptoms with restriction of function that cannot be further clarified by clinical examination or plain X-rays. Those affected usually display the so-called impingement syndrome with chronic shoulder pain (painful arc), which is usually the result of ruptures of the rotator cuff (Fig. 9.15.2) or of chronic inflammatory or degenerative processes of the articular soft tissues. Incomplete rupture of the rotator cuff unfortunately often eludes standard arthrographic demonstration. Loose bodies in the joint and adhesive capsulitis can, however, be clearly demonstrated arthrographically.

Chronic pain and restriction of movement in post-traumatic states in both growing and mature patients can be largely clarified by means of *arthrography of the elbow joint.* Examination of this joint is also indicated for demon-

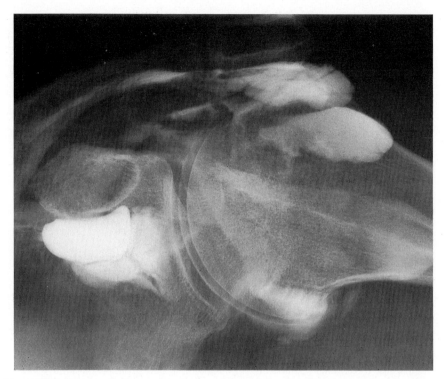

Fig. 9.15.2. Positive single-contrast arthrography of the shoulder joint (15 ml Iotrolan 300) in a 50-year-old patient after physical overtaxation. Diagnosis: complete rupture of the rotator cuff with contrast outlining the subacromial bursa and the subdeltoid bursa

strating loose bodies, mostly in osteochondritis dissecans with corresponding symptoms of "locking".

Injuries to the distal radioulnar articular cartilage ("triangular ligament") that result from radial fractures or from falling on the joint with a hyperextended hand often lead to painful conditions following immobilization, especially when the wrist is rotated. *With arthrography of the wrist,* rupture of the ligament can be superbly demonstrated (Fig. 9.15.3). Arthrography is also very useful in clarifying symptoms following chronic overuse of the wrist.

The primary indication for *arthrography of the ankle joint* (in almost 90% of cases) is acute trauma with deformity of the joint (Fig. 9.15.4). Capsular ligament ruptures without bone trauma can almost always be demonstrated in the acute stage. However, the films, for which the patient must remain in a fixed position, are often inconclusive. Due to the considerable pain, the examination cannot always be performed properly, and the risk of completely severing an already partially torn ligament through movement must not be forgotten.

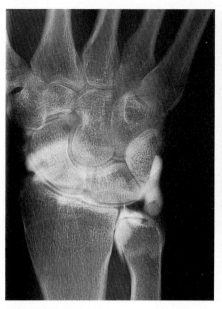

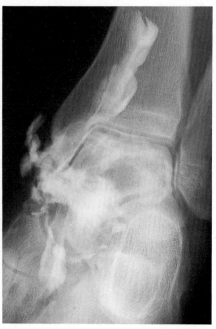

Fig. 9.15.3. Positive single-contrast arthrography of the wrist (5 ml Iotrolan 300) in a 26-year-old patient following gymnastics. Diagnosis: rupture of the distal radioulnar articular disc ("triangular ligament") with contrast imaging of the distal radioulnar joint

Fig. 9.15.4. Positive single-contrast arthrography of the ankle joint (5 ml Iotrolan 300) in a 33-year-old patient after a sports accident. Diagnosis: rupture of the deltoid ligament; spreading of the CM medially

For clarification of the condition of cartilage and bone in osteochondritis dissecans and in inflammatory, degenerative and post-traumatic articular changes with recurrent swelling, arthrography can be helpful.

In many paediatric radiology and paediatric orthopaedic centres, *arthrography of the hip joint* is used in hip dysplasia and Perthes' disease. The examination is less often performed on adults, however, there has been increasing success recently in clarifying cases of prosthesis loosening following endoprosthetic operations. Further important indications are coxitis and osteochondritis dissecans.

The arthrography of smaller joints is less frequent and only performed when a very specific problem is being investigated.

In summary, arthrography is the technique of choice in acute trauma or post-traumatic states, in inflammatory or degenerative processes of the articular soft tissues, in osteochondritis dissecans with or without loose bodies in the joint, and in the diagnosis of articular tumours.

Which Contrast Medium?

Arthrography makes unavoidable demands not only on the examiner's experience, competence and technique but also on the quality of the CM.

There are important requirements that an ideal X-ray CM should satisfy. In assessing CM quality, the most important criteria are: good and artefact-free contrast, optimal sharpness in outlining the various articular structures, good local tissue compatibility and general tolerability and slow absorption.

In historical terms, the development of orthographic technique since 1905 has been closely related to research and further development of CM. In the course of time, negative CM such as oxygen, carbon dioxide, air and positive oily and water-soluble X-ray CM were introduced in conjunction with single contrast and double-contrast technique.

The chemotoxicity of X-ray CM, the complications arising from negative or positive X-ray CM and from incorrect or careless administration, put a considerable burden on the method and hindered widespread clinical acceptance. It was not until the 1930s that radiologists had better tolerated water-soluble, ionic, tri-iodinated and X-ray CM at their disposal; these CM have adequately proven their reliability for over half a century.

The nonionic, monomeric, X-ray CM developed in the 1970s proved beneficial to arthrography, at a time when it was becoming an increasingly popular technique. The development of a dimeric, hexaiodinated, nonionic and water-soluble CM, Iotrolan 300, represents a significant further achievement in CM research; for over 2 years now, it has been the arthrographic CM preferred by many radiologists. This X-ray CM clearly permits a better and longer-lasting detailed demonstration of structures with very good contrast density and excellent image sharpness; it thus fulfils to a great extent the criteria listed above with excellent local and systemic tolerability [8]. The principal source of the superb qualities of this X-ray CM is its isotonicity with blood and body fluid. This minimizes the loss of contrast caused by the osmotically induced influx of fluid into the articular space.

Which Method?

Pneumarthrography, the single-contrast technique with negative CM, such as air, carbon dioxide or oxygen, is hardly ever still practiced, since the diagnostic quality is inadequate when compared to that of other techniques. It is performed, if at all, on patients with a known allergic diathesis [2].

Given the superb quality and tolerability of the nonionic X-ray CM available today and the effectiveness of prophylactic measures using H_1- and H_2-receptor blockers against undesirable side effects, little stands in the way of using positive X-ray CM for single contrast or double-contrast arthrography, even on patients theoretically at risk.

Approximately 20% of all arthrographies are performed with *single-contrast technique* and positive X-ray CM. With this technique, the amount of

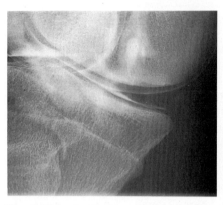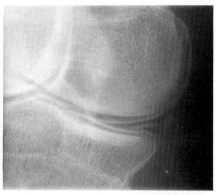

Fig. 9.15.5a, b. Positive single-contrast arthrography of the right knee joint (10 ml Iotrolan 300) in a 46-year-old patient with joint effusion following severe strain. Diagnosis immediately after CM administration without movement exercises, no lesion visible (**a**). A rupture of the meniscus is clearly depicted 10–15 min after CM administration and movement exercises (**b**)

CM appropriate to the given joint is administered free of air bubbles, intra-articularly and under fluoroscopic control. In the arthrography of smaller joints, 2–5 ml CM is given and in shoulder and knee-joint arthrography, ca. 10 ml or, in individual cases, more.

When the X-ray CM iotrolan is used as an arthrographic medium, joints have to be moved for a longer period of time to optimally distribute the administered CM and avoid misinterpretation (Fig. 9.15.5). Iotrolan has a higher viscosity than the other X-ray CM and thus requires correspondingly more time in order to outline natural or pathological folds, fissures and tears.

The most important advantages of the positive single-contrast technique are held to be its very good artefact-free sharpness of detail and high accuracy combined with an almost complete lack of impairment of joint function.

Double-contrast arthrography is the technique of choice of most examiners. It has proven its outstanding reliability particularly in the diagnosis of the shoulder and knee joint.

It is performed after controlled administration of positive X-ray CM under fluoroscopic control followed by gas/air insufflation. The amount of X-ray CM and gas varies considerably with both the joint and examiner involved. For the examination of the knee joint, 4–8 ml X-ray CM and 40–60 cm^3 air, carbon dioxide or oxygen are used. In shoulder arthrography, 3–5 ml X-ray CM and 10–15 cm^3 air or gas are quite sufficient.

The popularity of the double-contrast technique springs from its remarkably sharp contour definition and its "plastic" depiction of the individual articular structures. The disadvantages of the technique appear to be an increase in the risk of infection, greater irritation of the articular capsule, overshadowing effects due to foaming and an impairment of articular function after the examination.

General Rules Applicable to All Arthrographic Techniques

The following is a list of general rules that hold for all arthrographic procedures:
- Disinfect thoroughly, best by spraying and amply wetting the skin around the joint
- Shorten any troublesome hair growth at the point of injection with scissors, since shaving can injure the skin
- Cover the joint with a sterile slit towel
- Use sterile gloves
- Use sterile one-way syringes and cannulae
- Draw up the CM and the local anaesthetic into the syringe immediately prior to injection
- Avoid injecting at places where there are skin abrasions or inflammations
- Infiltration of anaesthetic is not obligatory in puncture of a joint. However, local anaesthesia is often appreciated by anxious patients
- Existing joint effusions should be largely drained (punctured) prior to CM administration if at all possible
- The intra-articular administration of CM and air should always occur under fluoroscopic control. Irritating CM extravasation into the articular soft tissues and consequent overshadowing effects can be avoided in this way
- Application of an adhesive absorbent dressing and/or compression bandage is required to protect the site of injection
- Thoroughly distribute the X-ray CM in the articular space by means of active and passive joint movements
- Take all films under fluoroscopic control
- Take concluding survey films of the entire joint. If necessary also obtain tomograms or computed tomograms.

Complications

Arthrography is quite a low-risk technique.

Local skin irritation caused by the disinfectant and sensitivity reactions to the local anaesthesia can occur, but they are relatively rare and not specific to this technique. An unpleasant "bubbling" sensation occurs only with the double-contrast technique, it is felt to be variably unpleasant by patients and can last up to 36 h [3].

Soft tissue emphysema following faulty gas insufflation can be painful and last up to 2 days. Very unusual complications such as pneumomediastinum and air embolism are described in the literature. They may be viewed as special and isolated cases related to faulty technique on the part of the operator.

Small reactive effusions and accompanying feelings of articular tension or worsening of existing symptoms and synovial irritation are difficult to explain aetiologically. On the one hand, they can be taken to be reactions to the X-ray CM; this appears improbable, however, given the good local tolerability of modern nonionic X-ray CM. On the other hand, they could be induced by the intensive stress manoeuvres during the examination.

Local infection and bacterial arthritis should not occur if the rules of cleanliness and asepsis are strictly followed. Lindblom [5] mentions two cases of arthritis out of 4000 cases, Wirth et al. [10], one incident of staphylococcal arthritis in a diabetic, whereas we did not experience a single case of articular infection in our total test group of 14000 arthrographies.

Occurrence of systemic allergic reactions, such as urticaria with itching, oedema of the eyelids, feelings of unease, and circulatory instability may be associated with the use of ionic and nonionic X-ray CM. In ca. 2000 arthrographies with the dimeric, hexaiodinated, nonionic, X-ray CM Iotrolan 300, eight patients complained of similar symptoms 8 h after the examination. With oral antihistamines, symptoms were quickly terminated. Only in one case were corticosteroids also administered. It is worth noting that in some of these cases CM hypersensitivity was known to exist.

Lethal complications have not been described as yet in the literature. Newberg et al. in a statistical summary of 126,000 cases [6] noted 317 local and systemic complications, but not a single fatality following arthrography.

Prospects

Arthrography – due to its diagnostic power and its high rate of accuracy – retains its status as one of the most important techniques for the study of joints. Incomprehensibly, in many places, especially in the United States, arthroscopy has resulted in a marked decline in arthrographic examinations. Responsible orthopaedic surgeons and trauma specialists, however, are aware of the limits of arthroscopy as a diagnostic technique and employ endoscopic techniques almost solely for therapeutic purposes. In our own experience, most patients who come for arthrography have been referred by precisely those physicians who themselves perform arthroscopic procedures. Nonspecific postoperative symptoms are also monitored primarily arthrographically.

Neither arthroscopy (Fig. 9.15.6) nor CT (Fig. 9.15.7) and US, when viewed critically and objectively, can completely replace arthrography. Only MRI can be seen as representing a truly competitive technique; however, MRI is time-consuming and costly and cannot be employed in routine examinations in every institution [4].

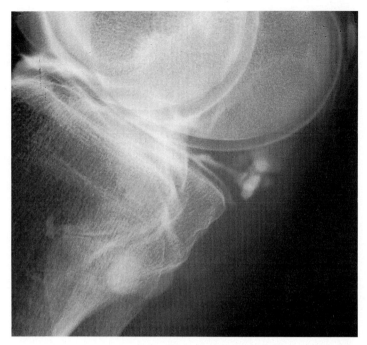

Fig. 9.15.6. Positive single-contrast arthrography of the left knee joint (10 ml Iotrolan 300) in a 52-year-old patient who had already suffered long-term symptoms and undergone arthroscopy without findings. Diagnosis: old horizontal rupture of the medial posterior horn with intracapsular ganglion

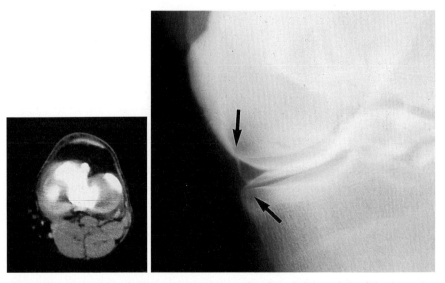

Fig. 9.15.7a, b. Positive single-contrast arthrography of the left knee joint (10 ml Iotrolan 300) in a 41-year-old patient after a sports accident and CT without findings (**a**). Diagnosis: vertical longitudinal rupture of the medial posterior horn (**b**)

References

1. Annewanter G (1984) Die Meniscusläsion dargestellt im Arthrogramm und ihre Korrelation zum Operationspräparat. Inaugural dissertation, Free University of Berlin
2. Dalinka MK (1980) Arthrography. Springer, Berlin Heidelberg New York
3. Freiberger RH, Killoran PJ, Gardona G (1966) Arthrography of the knee by double contrast method. Am J Roentgenol 97:736–747
4. Hall FM (1987) Arthrography, past, present and future. AJR 149:561–562
5. Lindblom K (1948) Arthrography of the knee, a roentgenographic and anatomical study. Acta Radiol Suppl 74 (Stockh)
6. Newberg AH, Munn CS, Robbins AH (1985) Complications of arthrography. Radiology 155:605–606
7. Richlin P, Rüttimann A, Del Buono MS (1971) Meniscus lesions. Practical Problems of clinical diagnosis – Arthrography and Therapy. Grune and Stratton, New York
8. Schmidt M, Papassotiriou V (1989) Arthrography with iotrolan. In: Taenzer V, Wende S (eds) Recent developments in nonionic contrast media. Thieme, Stuttgart, pp 182–189
9. Scholz J, Weyrauch U (1981) Korrelation zwischen Arthrographie und Operationsbefund bei Meniscusläsionen. Z Orthop 119:177–181
10. Wirth W, Mihicic J (1989) Arthrographie. In: Schinz (ed) Radiologische Diagnostik in Klinik und Praxis, VI/1. Thieme, Stuttgart, p 293

9.16 What Advantages Do Nonionic Contrast Media Have for Paediatric Patients?

H. J. Kaufmann and *C. Bassir*

In this section experience accumulated to date with nonionic CM in paediatric patients will be evaluated. The first nonionic CM to be used was Amipaque and in the past 10 years experience has been gained with the newer agents allowing a number of conclusions can be reached.

The different areas of application of CM will be analysed, with some comments on recognizable benefits to the patient. We are, of course, aware of the cost/benefit problem; however, this will not be of major concern here since one further argument for the use of these new agents in the paediatric patient, besides its superior tolerance, is "the younger the patient, the smaller the amount needed".

We would like to stress that ionic CM still have a somewhat limited but definite place, e.g. micturating cystourethrography (MCU), still a relatively frequently requested investigation, and imaging of the genital tract, where there is no present justification for the use of the more expensive nonionic CM.

What major advantages can now be recognized?

Intravenous Urography

The most striking improvement after the introduction of monomeric non-ionic CM available in ready-to-use form was a completely transformed atmosphere and attitude in the examination room for i.v. urography, angiography and/or CT. Whereas in the past restlessness of the patient, hives, itching urticarial rash and, quite often, vomiting were encountered in significantly high incidence, such phenomena are now strikingly unusual. This means that the tension that existed prior to, during and after the administration of ionic CM has been replaced by an atmosphere free of fear and anxiety. A review of over 10 000 paediatric i.v. urographies performed by paediatric radiologists in Germany did not reveal a single case of major complication.

Computed Tomography Examination

Another significant improvement has come about in the performance of contrast-enhanced CT examinations. Better imaging studies with fewer motion artefacts are the result of hardly any restlessness or motion during the injection. The intravenous cannula must be in place before the patient is brought into the examination room.

Contrast Media Extravasation

A minor argument, but certainly not one to be overlooked, for the use of nonionic CM is supported by the observation that extravasation of ionic CM may lead to local necrosis. In young children veins may easily perforate with a considerable leak of CM into the adjacent soft tissues. During bolus injection, with or without a pressure injector, major extravasation may occur. Whereas in the days of nonionic CM surgical intervention was recommended, this is no longer the case.

Gastrointestinal Tract

Major advances have come about in the use of nonionic CM for gastrointestinal examinations in newborns and infants [12]. We have accumulated results from well over 600 such examinations using the newly developed compounds.

In our latest study we evaluated the acceptance and tolerance of a new isotonic, nonionic substance, Iotrolan (Isovist-300), in newborns and babies and the quality of the examinations obtained.

From May 1988 to August 1990 we performed 133 examinations, among these six premature infants and ten children with an age of less than 1 week. Currently, the following CM for gastrointestinal examinations were available:

1. Barium sulfate suspension
2. Ionic iodinated water-soluble CM
3. Nonionic monomeric iodinated water-soluble CM
4. Nonionic dimeric iodinated water-soluble CM.

Barium suspensions are contraindicated if aspiration, perforation or intestinal obstruction is suspected. Aspiration of strongly hyperosmolar ionic iodinated CM (osmolality about 1500–2150 mosm/kg at 37°C) can produce a potentially life-threatening pulmonary oedema. There is now hardly any danger using nonionic iodinated CM (osmolality about 630 mosm/kg at 37°C) but, if iso-osmolality is required (aspiration/perforation) they can only be used diluted at 150 mg I/ml. The major advantage of iotrolan is its iso-osmolality with blood (320 mosm/kg), so that an iodine concentration of 300 mg I/ml is available at blood osmolality. It seems that the only disadvantage of iotrolan is its high price, but considering of its advantages and the small volumes required in newborns and babies, this should not be a major obstacle.

Conclusion

This new CM offers the following advantages:
1. Since it is iso-osmolar it can be used without dilution
2. Due to its sweet taste its acceptance is excellent and no additive is required
3. Due to its six iodine atoms per molecule high iodine concentrations may be achieved in low osmolality solutions
4. If it reaches the trachea, pleura or peritoneum no ill effects has so far been recognized
5. Distal small bowel and the large bowel are well visualized due to a lack of osmotic dilution. No water or electrolytes are drawn into the lumen
6. Unlike barium, it presents no problem to the surgeon if after a contrast study the operative procedure requires opening of a part of the gastrointestinal tract.

With the possibility now of performing contrast studies in practically all of their applications even in newborns and premature babies, irrespective of the severity of their clinical condition, the spectrum of indications could be markedly extended. This is the result of the far better tolerance of the nonionic CM by the immature infant. Paediatricians, neonatologists and particularly also paediatric surgeons may be assured that by this approach better diagnostic and therapeutic management of even the youngest, smallest and most severely affected paediatric patients be achieved.

Thyroid and Iodinated Contrast Media

Contrary to observations in the adult patient, even after large CM doses no cases of thyrotoxicosis have been recorded during infancy. After angiocardiography small babies – especially neonates – should be monitored for the possibility of hypothyroidism. This response could be the result of small amounts of free iodide in the CM. Hypothyroidism after small amounts of CM – 1–2 ml for the demonstration of patency and location of central venous catheters – has also been observed. The determination of TSH, T_3 and T_4 1 week after a CM study is recommended by Grüters et al. [3].

Conclusion

At a round-table discussion at the Florence Meeting of the European Society of Paediatric Radiology it was decided that patients of paediatric age should have the benefit of the nonionic CM for intravascular studies. The great advantages of these agents in gastrointestinal studies of babies and infants was recognized and stressed. A very powerful argument is consideration of the subjective discomfort of infants and children having to undergo studies with CM. Where the welfare of our children is concerned, cost consciousness cannot be a valid argument against these considerations.

References

1. Cohen MD (1982) Prolonged visualization of the gastrointestinal tract with metrizamide. Radiology 143:327–328
2. Cohen MD, Smith WL, Smith JA et al. (1980) The use of metrizamide (Amipaque) to visualize the gastrointestinal tract in children: a preliminary report. Clin Radiol 31:635–641
3. Grüters A, l'Allemand D, Klett M, Helge H (1987) The problem of the influence of modern iodinated contrast media on thyroid metabolism in babies. In: Kaufmann HJ (ed) Contrast media in pediatric radiology. Schering AG, Berlin, pp 87–90

9.17 What Is the Role of Newer Contrast Media in Interventional Radiology?

P. Dawson

CM are used in most fluoroscopically guided interventional procedures. Such procedures may be categorized in two groups – vascular and nonvascular. In the nonvascular procedures, such as hepatobiliary, urogenital, etc., though large total doses may be used, intravasation is slow and most of the CM will be passed out via the gut or the bladder. High dose toxicity is very rarely a problem, therefore. It is true that anaphylactoid reactions may occasionally occur in such procedures but these are rare. Nevertheless, there is a case for using nonionic agents to reduce this risk even further in such patients with significantly increased risk factors but this case is weaker than when CM is administered intravascularly.

Angiographic interventional procedures are a different matter because the CM enters the circulation immediately. Nonionic agents should be used in patients with definable risk factors as in any diagnostic procedure. Considerable total doses may be used in complex angiographic interventional procedures and it is in this context that the nonionic agents come into their own. Low osmolalities, low chemotoxicities and zero sodium content make them most suitable for use in procedures anticipated to entail a high total dose [1].

There has been some debate about the ideal CM for use in the specific case of angioplasty. Low osmolality media (ionic or nonionic) have generally been used to minimize pain of the concomitant angiography and, it has also been argued, to minimize endothelial injury. This last point seems unconvincing since the endothelial injury caused by *any* CM is likely to be swamped by the gross mechanical or thermal injury caused by the procedure itself.

Some are now arguing that nonionic low osmolality agents should not be used because they have weak anticoagulant and antiplatelet properties as compared with the ionic agents [2]. This also seems a rather spurious argument in this context because any "anticoagulant" injected locally will have only a very transient effect. Much more important is likely to be the patient's state of systemic anticoagulation. The use of adequate systemic heparinization seems likely, therefore, to be much more important [2]. In coronary angioplasty, in particular, it would seem a pity to throw away the advantage of a proven, distinctly low cardiotoxicity as offered by nonionic agents in order to chase a theoretical anticoagulant gain.

All this being said, no clinical trial comparing the outcome of angioplasty, short or longer term, with different CM has, as yet, been reported, so it must be said that the jury is still out.

References

1. Dawson P, Hemingway AP (1987) Contrast agent doses in interventional radiology. J Intervent Radiol 2:145–146
2. Dawson P, Strickland NH (1991) Thromboembolic phenomena in clinical angiography. Role of materials and technique. J Vasc Intervent Radiol 2:125–135

CHAPTER 10

Contrast Media for Magnetic Resonance Imaging and Ultrasound

10.1 Contrast Media for Clinical Magnetic Resonance Imaging

H. P. Niendorf and *J. C. Dinger*

The substances most suitable as CM for MRI are those that change the relaxation times of the anatomic structures to be depicted. Both paramagnetic and superparamagnetic substances are appropriate for this purpose. The magnetic moments of the individual atoms or molecules of paramagnetic substances point randomly outside a magnetic field. When an external magnetic field is applied, they align themselves in such a way that, as a whole, an "induced" magnetic field parallel to the external one arises that increases linearly in strength proportional to the strength of the external field. Superparamagnetic substances are microscopically small (Fe_3O_4 < 0.035 µm in diameter), solid particles, in which even outside of a magnetic field the magnetic moments of the individual atoms or molecules are parallel in alignment as a result of the forces between these particles. The resulting magnetic moments of the individual particles are independently aligned when outside of a magnetic field. Since these magnetic moments align in parallel in an external magnetic field, a strongly induced magnetic field arises when such a field is applied. Initially, it grows linearly in strength proportional to the strength of the external field. However, as the strength of the latter increases, the strength of the induced field begins to grow more slowly as equilibrium is approached.

On the basis of the strongly induced magnetic field, superparamagnetic substances in the smallest quantities will influence signal intensity; nevertheless, paramagnetic substances can be utilized more flexibly, since they can be administered to the body in aqueous solutions. Superparamagnetic substances are administered as suspensions whose particles are phagocystosed by the reticuloendothelial system (RES) when they are given intravascularly. Other substances, such as ferromagnetics, have only limited suitability as CM, or none at all.

Of the experimentally tested paramagnetic CM, those compounds containing gadolinium have been studied most. Gadolinium diethylenetriamine penta-acetic acid (gadolinium-DTPA; Magnevist), which was the first paramagnetic CM authorized for cranial and spinal MRI in West Germany, the United States, and Japan (in 1988), is the only substance today that is available worldwide.

Gadolinium-DTPA

The effect of the extremely hydrophilic and low-viscosity complex gadolinium-DPTA on signal intensity is largely determined by the paramagnetic metal, gadolinium (Gd), whereas the pharmacokinetic qualities of the complex are determined by DTPA, a substance well known from nuclear medicine. As in every chelate complex, in aqueous solution a definite part of the complex dissociates into metal ion (Gd^{3+}) and ligand ($DTPA^{5-}$). The dissociation constant for Gd-DTPA lies between 10^{-22} and 10^{-23}; thus, there is an extreme shift in the equilibrium of the dissociation reaction in the direction of the undissociated complex. This high stability guarantees that free metal ions are not produced in quantities affecting tolerance.

Gd-DTPA spreads itself over almost the entire extracellular space (EDS). There is no indication of its passage into intracellular space to any significant degree. Owing to its molecular size and strong hydrophilicity, the complex is also not able to pass through an intact blood-brain barrier. A damaged blood-brain barrier, however, is permeable for Gd-DTPA and is thus highly sensitive to detection in this way. Since damage to the blood-brain barrier is not directly detectable by means of conventional MRI, the use of Gd-DTPA often offers the possibility of providing clinically relevant diagnostic information. The speed and degree of increase in signal intensity is dependent here on the extent of damage. The degree of vascularization of the investigated region and the size of the interstitial space, i.e. the number of water molecules whose relaxation times are influencable by Gd-DTPA, also play a part here. The difference in signal intensity (contrast) between a definite area and its surroundings are also contingent upon the point of time of measurement, the parameters chosen for imaging and the signal intensity of the surroundings.

In the usual clinical dosage (0.1 mmol/kg body weight), the body receives, in spite of the ionic character of Gd-DTPA, only a small quantity of osmotically active particles (ca. 20 mosm). This is clearly less than in an X-ray examination with nonionic, iodinated, X-ray CM (e.g. 58 mosm pro 100 ml iohexol; 350 mg I/ml). The half-life of the substance, which is excreted unchanged by glomerular filtration, is ca. 90 min [10].

Despite its exemplary tolerability (see below), Gd-DTPA should not be used as a matter of course. It is always indicated if CNS lesions (e.g. tumours, metastases, infections, leptomeningeal lesions, active multiple sclerosis lesions) are to be discovered or excluded, or better defined or more precisely characterized. Moreover, it can also be indicated for patients whose general condition warrants avoiding long imaging times with T_2-weighted sequences. If, however, numerous metastases are already known about from conventional imaging, it is generally of only limited clinical value to detect further metastases. Frequently, one also forgoes contrast-enhanced MRI when excluding tumours, if the T_2-weighted images appear normal and there is no strong clinical suspicion. However, in a series of well-known cases, lesions became detectable only after Gd-DTPA was administered.

The optimal doses with which it is possible to achieve sufficient contrast depictable lesions is considered to be 0.1 mmol Gd-DTPA per kg body weight [7] In borderline cases, the first administration can be followed within 30 min by a further injection of 0.1 mmol/kg body weight. As a rule, the MRI images can be made from 0 to 45 min after CM administration. For the visualization of hypophyseal microadenoma, it is necessary to start making images immediately, since after CM administration the hypodense lesion can only be reliably distinguished from the strongly hyperdense, normal hypophyseal tissue from a short period of time.

In any individual case, the pulse sequence most suitable is contingent upon the technical equipment at the operator's disposal; however, Gd-DTPA, when indicated, is in principle suitable for all clinically used types of magnets and instruments. Heavily T_1-weighted spin-echo sequences are preferable for optimal anatomical visualization. However, if minimal examination time is an issue (e.g. in dynamic examination), heavily T_1-weighted gradient echo sequences are more suitable [5].

Tolerance

Data exist from a total of 15 593 subjects and patients from phase IV clinical tests, in which adverse effects were noted according to a standardized protocol [6]. If one disregards local sensations of warmth at the site of injection, adverse effects were observed in about 1% of the patients; in patients with a history of allergies this rose to 2.6%. None of the effects observed in these studies was life-threatening. The spectrum of adverse effects is qualitatively very comparable to that of iodinated, nonionic, X-ray CM. Moreover, the overall rate of adverse effects following the intravenous injection of 0.1 or 0.2 mmol Gd-DTPA/kg body weight is two to three times lower.

No correlation between age (including the 2- to 18-year-old age group) and frequency of adverse effects was observed. Accordingly, in CNS indications, the preparation is authorized for use in all age groups of 2 years and above. After current clinical tests are concluded, the manufacturer will seek to have this authorization extended to cover the newborn and infants.

For reasons of safety, injection rate was limited to 10 ml/min in early clinical studies. After wide-ranging experience with bolus injections [3] and with doses of up to 0.2 mmol/kg body weight now available, there is no longer any justification for this limitation.

The very small number of spontaneous side effects reported after its authorization provides even further support for the markedly favorable side-effect profile of the drug. In over 5.000.000 administrations, adverse effects were reported in less fewer than 0.03% of the cases [12]. Even if one assumes that the actual overall number is an order of magnitude higher, these figures still reflect very good tolerance data in clinical tests. Regardless of the statistics, it is certain that the registration of life-threatening incidents is much more complete. Here we find two cases of glottic oedema, six of anaphylactoid shock, one of intracerebral haemorrhage, and four deaths, all reported in temporal connection with the administration of Gd-DTPA (as of 31 October 1990). The intracerebral haemorrhage and the four deaths did not result from anaphylactoid reactions, and in the estimation of investigators cannot be causally related to the CM administration. Nonetheless, it has become clear that Gd-DTPA can produce – even if only extremely rarely – anaphylactoid reactions. For this reason, it should be a basic policy not to perform contrast-enhanced MRI tests unless emergency care is guaranteed in terms of both personnel and equipment.

Gd-DTPA in diagnostic doses demonstrates, regardless of any pre-existing renal insufficiency, no effects on serum creatinine levels or other indicators of kidney function. Depending on the degree of restriction of function the excretion phase may be slightly longer. In addition, in patients with renal failure, Gd-DTPA can easily be removed from the body by dialysis. As an example, its half-life in patients with a Fresenius F60 membrane haemodialyser is of the same magnitude (1.87 h ± 0.71 h) as in patients with healthy kidneys and without haemodialysis [4].

Not Yet Authorized Indications for Gd-DTPA

In some countries Gd-DTPA is now authorized for use also outside the CNS. Gd-DTPA has proven useful in a variety of other clinical conditions: for example, in the exclusion of malignant diseases of the female breast in diagnostically difficult cases – according to all experience, carcinomas always show an increase in signal intensity following Gd-DTPA administration [2]. Thus, the lack of such an increase has to be interpreted to indicate the exclusion of carcinoma. Moreover, this CM appears to improve the visualization of myocardial infarction, reperfusion after fibrinolysis and the infiltration depth of Pancoast's tumour.

The differential diagnosis of focal lesions in liver and spleen and the detection, differentiation and differential diagnosis of lesions in the area of the kidneys and adrenal glands can be improved with Gd-DTPA. It also appears to make possible the semiquantitative, incidental determination of renal function and to provide evidence of kidney transplant organ rejection in cases of poor renal function. Contrast-enhanced imaging is especially well suited for the diagnosis of endometrial carcinoma of the uterus in gynaecological tumours. Easier discovery of lesions, better estimation of the extent of tumour, better distinction of fluid in the uterine cavity and necrosis, and more precise tumour staging [1]. In the extremities, for example, necrosis and oedema of tumour tissue can be better distinguished and detection of postoperative tumour recurrence can be greatly improved.

The hard connective tissue of joint capsules, ligaments, and menisci has no "signal" due to a lack of mobile hydrogen atomprotons. In MRI, these structures are imaged indirectly by contrast with surrounding structures such as synovium or fat. The articular cartilage also provides relatively low signal.

Because of the small differences in contrast among these articular structures, they cannot always be satisfactorily differentiated in conventional imaging; the chronic changes of the articular cartilage in rheumatic disease are inadequately depicted. A positive CM such as Gd-DTPA that, on intraarticular injection, improves indirect imaging by increasing the signal intensity of the synovium can make it easier to differentiate between structures. Clinical tests have shown that even small cartilage defects can be detected with Gd-DTPA in a concentration of 2 mmol/1. Gradient echo sequences in combination with Gd-DTPA appear to be the most suitable way to depict these changes.

MRI does not always satisfactorily differentiate intra-abdominal organs and pathological lesions from intestinal loops. For this purpose, a special formulation of Gd-DTPA has been developed, containing 1 mmol Gd-DTPA and 15 g/l of the hexavalent sugar alcohol mannitol. The CM is administered orally or rectally. For the upper gastrointestinal tract the dose is at least 300 ml; if the entire gastrointestinal tract is to be imaged, the dose can be increased up to 1000 ml. Rectally, between 20 and 500 ml is given. In a clinical test, side effects were observed in 11 of 183 patients (6%). Ten of these cases involved mild gastrointestinal symptoms such as flatulence and watery stools, which can be attributed to the bacterial decomposition of mannitol or the administration of large volumes of liquid. None of the 11 patients required treatment.

Gd-DTPA – in the above formulation, even in T_2-weighted sequences – always demonstrates a positive contrast effect. Both normal pancreas and one which is inflamed or contains a tumour can be better distinguished from stomach and duodenum, and intestinal loops can be better differentiated from surrounding tumour (e.g. lymphoma). Image artefacts and increased signal noise that arise through movements of the positive CM-filled intestine can be adequately repressed by glucagon. Spin-echo sequences with short repetition and echo times can reduce the image-degrading influences of breathing and heart action. Though Gd-DTPA produces better intestine-tumour contrast than negative CM (see below), the opposite is the case in intestine-abdominal fat tissue contrast. Nevertheless, even in the latter case, sufficient contrast is possible with T_2-weighted sequences [1].

Other Paramagnetic, Extracellular Space Markers

The clinical development of a series of other Gd chelates is not yet complete. Thus it is not possible to confidently assess them. These chelates spread through extracellular spaces (ECS) and their half-lives or plasma concentrations are not different from those of Gd-DTPA in any clinically relevant way. Tolerance will be a decisive factor in the choice of CM once further GD chelates are authorized. It is not immediately clear that a direct analogy to the ionic and nonionic X-ray CM can be made here, i.e. that the electrically neutral preparations Gd-DTPA-BMA, Gd-DO3A-HP and Gd-DTPA bismorpholid will prove to be better tolerated. First of all, though these substances are electrically neutral towards the outside, the coordinating bonds of the central gadolinium atom with the ligands have more of an ionic character. Secondly, even in ionic preparations, the physidogical stress produced by osmotically active particles is very small. The ECS markers Gd-DOTA, Bd-DO3A-HP, Gd-DTPA bismorpholid and Gd-DTPA-BMA are of similar stability to Gd-DTPA. Existing differences in stability are more of a theoretical nature, since all of the substances produce only very small quantities of free metal ions when administered in diagnostic doses.

Paramagnetic Contrast Media for Imaging the Intravascular Space and the Liver

For certain clinical problems, blood pool rather than extracellular space markers are needed. An intravascular space marker could be utilized, for example, for the quantitative determination of myocardial perfusion; it could thus combine the functional diagnosis provided by the methods of nuclear medicine with the high resolving power of MRI. To prevent a paramagnetic CM from passing into the interstitial tissues from normal blood vessels without the blood-brain barrier, it is necessary to have molecules that are of greater size than the Gd chelates described above. This can be accomplished by binding Gd-DTPA to such substances as albumin, dextran, or polylysine. In this way, it has been possible in animal experiments to make good-quality images of arteries and veins with diameters of less than 1 mm [11]. Such markers also appear suitable for direct and indirect lymphography. It is also conceivable that substances of specific molecular size could be developed which, except in haemorrhage, only pass into ECS in cases of increased capillary permeability, e.g. in inflammation and tumours; this would make it possible to detect such lesions.

There are basically two strategies for the specific, contrast-enhanced imaging of the liver: CM is concentrated in either RES or in the hepatocytes. The first approach is based upon phagocytosis of small particles; in the second, hepatobiliary CM are taken up by the hepatic cells by diffusion or by transport proteins and subsequently excreted into the intestine via the bile (this makes contrast imaging of the bile ducts perhaps also possible). Paramagnetic CM such as Mn-DTPA or Gd-BOPTA are potential candidates as hepatobiliary CM. For precise assessment, one will need to await further clinical development of these substances.

In order to have paramagnetic chelates such as Gd-DTPA phagocytosed, one can encapsulate them in liposomes. Liposomes consist of bimolecular lipid lamellae that spontaneously form small hollow spheres. The size and wall thickness of the liposomes influence the CM action and pharmokinetics of these vesicles. In animal experiments, strong parenchyma-lesion contrast in liver and spleen can be attained with liposomes containing

Gd chelates and, on the basis of their relatively long half-lives in the blood, they are also partially suitable as blood-pool markers. The results of the first human-pharmacological studies should be available soon.

Superparamagnetic Contrast Media

Superparamagnetic substances, unlike paramagnetic substances, are always solids that are introduced into the body as suspensions rather than in aqueous solutions. For MRI, different iron oxide compounds (ferrite and magnetite) have been developed, which are usually coated with dextran or a dextran derivative. After intravenous injection, they are phagocytosed by RES (see liposomes above); due to their sharp reduction of T_2 relaxation time, they trigger a signal in healthy hepatic tissue. In contrast, tumours and lesions that do not possess any RES present untransformed images. Tumours with RES activity or residual RES activity, however, continue to be subject to a signal-reducing effect. Superparamagnetic substances are extraordinarily effective CM, inducing strong signal changes even in the smallest concentrations. Nevertheless, it is pharmaceutically difficult and costly to produce particles of appropriate size with largely constant diameters. Moreover, in animal experiments, though many of these compounds in intravenous administration show a high LD_{50}, they also demonstrate marked adverse cardiovascular effects. AMI 25 has been subject to the greatest testing. It consists of dextran-coated Fe_2O_3/Fe_3O_4 particles with a diameter from 0.5 to 1.0 µm. Its half-life in blood is 15 min [9]. Its elimination from the RES varies widely. Its half-life in human liver is about 8 days [8]. In clinical studies, 10–50 µmol iron per kilogram body weight was injected, where the rapid injection of 40 µmol/kg relatively often led to persisting hypotension. In smaller doses, which are probably also sufficient for diagnosis, these effects have as yet not been observed. The advantage of superparamagnetic CM resides in their ability to lower minimal resolution size, such as in the case of small metastases. Due to be described difficulties, however, it is unclear whether superparamagnetic CM containing iron oxide well be approved for use in the near future. Perhaps the undesirable effects can be eliminated in part or even in full through small changes in formulation.

Similarly to Gd chelates, particulate iron oxides can be used as enteral CM. They lead to continuing signal loss in the entire gastrointestinal tract. They cause less signal noise than Gd-DTPA (see above) and make possible high contrast between the intestine and bordering abdominal fat. The demarcation of the intestinal wall per se is poorer than with Gd-DTPA. Both diarrhoea and a sensation of bloatedness have been reported as undesirable results following the administration of CM containing iron oxide. Presently it is not possible to make a sufficiently reliable cost-benefit analysis of such substances.

In terms of future developments, the greatest advances should come from specific CM (e.g. liposomes containing CM, superparamagnetic and polymeric paramagnetic substances). As compared with the very well tolerated Gd-DTPA, only minimal progress in the development of nonspecific ECS markers can be expected in the near future.

References

1. Hamm B, Laniado M, Saini S (1990) Contrast-enhanced magnetic resonance imaging of the abdomen and the pelvis. Magn Reson Q 6:108–135
2. Heywang SH (1990) Gd-DTPA-enhanced MRI of the breast. In: Bydder G (eds) Contrast media in MRI. Medicom Europe, Bussum, pp 261–265
3. Kashanian FK, Goldstein HA, Blumetti RF et al (1990) Rapid bolus injection of gadopentetate dimeglumine: absence of side effects in normal volunters. AJNR 11:853–856
4. Lackner K, Krahe T, Götz R et al (1990) The dialysability of Gd-DTPA. In: Bydder G (eds) Contrast media in MRI. Medicom Europe, Bussum, pp 321–326
5. Laniado M, Niendorf HP, Schörner W et al (1986) Spin echo and inversion recovery sequences for gadolinium-DTPA enhanced magnetic resonance imaging of intracranial tumors. Acta Radiol (Suppl) 369:469–471
6. Niendorf HP, Dinger JC, Haustein J et al (1990) Tolerance of Gd-DTPA: clinical experience. In: Bydder G (eds) Contrast media in MRI. Medicom Europe, Bussum, pp 31–39
7. Niendorf HP, Laniado M, Semmler W et al (1987) Dose administration of gadolinium-DTPA in MR imaging of intracranial tumors. Am J Neuroradiol 8:803–815
8. Saini S, Stark DD, Hahn PF et al (1989) Are superparamagnetic ferrite particles cleared from the liver? Radiology 173:175
9. Stark DD, Weissleder R, Elizondo G et al (1988) Superparamagnetic iron oxide: clinical application as a contrast agent for magnetic resonance imaging of the liver. Radiology 168:297–301
10. Weinmann HJ, Laniado M, Mützel W (1984) Pharmacokinetics of gadolinium-DTPA/dimeglumine after intravenous injection into healthy volunteers. Physiol Chem Phys Med NMR 16:167–172
11. Weinmann HJ, Press WR, Radüchel B et al (1990) Characteristics of Gd-DTPA and new derivatives. In: Bydder G (eds) Contrast media in MRI. Medicom Europe, Bussum, pp 19–30
12. Niendorf HP, Haustein J, Clauss W, Cornelius I (1993) Safety and risk of gadolinium-DTPA: Extended clinical experience after more than 5.000,000 applications. Advances in MRI Contrast 1993; 2:12–19

10.2 Ultrasonographic Contrast Media

R. Schlief, R. Schürmann, and *H. P. Niendorf*

Introduction

In US imaging, the intensity of echo signals and thus the contrast are dependent upon the character of the acoustic backscattering in the region being examined. It is known that there are two physically different qualities of the echoes from an examined area. On the one hand, elastic US waves are reflected from those boundary surfaces that are much larger than the wavelengths (ca. 0.3–1.0 mm), e.g. from organ boundaries. On the other hand, dispersal echoes (internal echoes) and overlapping patterns (texture) arise in anatomical structures that are smaller than the incident wavelengths. Aside from the reflecting lines of the organ boundaries, these differences in the overall echo signal intensity ("echogenicity") of a region and its texture also result in the demarcation of anatomical structures in the examined region ("contrast").

For this reason, all media that have an echogenicity or texture distinct from that of body tissue can, in principle, be used as "contrast media". "Hypoechoic CM" can facilitate the recognition of echogenic boundary surfaces. For example, filling the cavity of uterus with a physiological saline solution can facilitate the assessment of the endometrium or the location of myomas. However, the basic disadvantages of hypoechoic or nonechoic CM are their lack of specificity (i.e. echoes could also be missing for other reasons) and the fact that they fail to visualize movement and flow phenomena, such as vascular blood flow. For this reason, one usually takes "echo CM" to mean signal-enhancing media or *echogenic CM*. Only echogenic CM enable flow phenomena to be directly observed in B scanning. Doppler signals to be intensified, or CM to be used as an indicator solution for determining function (e.g. contrast-enhanced hysterosalpingosonography; visualization of cardiovascular shunt flows; cardiac output from the curve of CM dilution).

The development of reproducibly echogenic CM took longer than was initially expected. The necessity of developing a preparation that contains physiologically degradable acoustic scatterers in micrometre dimensions was one important reason for this.

It has been common knowledge since the pioneering work of Gramiak and Shah [6] and Meltzer et al. [8] that tiny gas bubbles ("microbubbles") are very effective US scatterers. They are in fact the echogenically active components of the agitated, injected solutions used in cardiology. All currently known industrial developments of echo-enhancing CM are ultimately based upon microbubbles [11]. Due to their special acoustic properties, the part played by microbubbles in US CM is similar in importance to that of iodine in X-ray CM or Gadolinium in MRI CM.

Without the addition of stabilizing aids, the short life-span of such microbubbles poses a basic problem. The lack of stability is a primary source of the inability to reproduce reliably individually developed echo-enhancing CM. Even greater bubble stability is required to achieve passage through the pulmonary capillary vessels. To date, published data report only two preparations in clinical development in which this degree of stability has been achieved, and with which, following intravenous injection, the echo signal is enhanced even in the left ventricle and the systemic arterial vascular bed (Albunex and a Schering AG trial drug designated as SH U 508 A).

Types and State of Development of Echogenic CM

The echogenic CM currently being used or clinically tested can be divided into three physically different types, each representing a different principle of microbubble stabilization.

Liquids Containing Microbubbles ("Microfoam")

The oldest known contrast administration technique involves the use of agitated or foamed injection solutions to produce echogenic effects in the blood during echocardiographic examinations. The first publication describing this effect appeared as early as 1968 [6]. In the following years, various injectable solutions were investigated as possible transport media for increasing contrast and in vivo life-span. Various preparatory techniques were also compared (shaking; foaming under a three-way tap; foaming with US high energy, i.e. "sonification"). In several papers the superiority of the sonification method was shown in regard to bubble dimensions and the intensity of CM effect; however, it has not yet been possible to produce microbubbles in a purely liquid suspension that are reproducible and stable enough to warrant being designated as injectable CM. An in vivo stability sufficient for attaining diagnostically relevant contrast effects after passage through pulmonary capillaries has yet to be achieved. For this reason, the use of CM of this type remains limited to venous vessels, the right ventricle and body cavities.

Hollow Gas-Filled Microspheres

With the help of a special sonification technique and by using human albumin as a solution medium, it has been possible to produce air-filled microspheres that survive pulmonary capillary passage and produce left-ventricle contrast effects. Individual preparations are cited in the literature [9], but the industrial development of this type of echogenic CM is represented only by Albunex [5]. The preparation is being clinically developed in the United States (Molecular Biosystems, Mallinckrodt), Europe (Nycomed) and Japan (Shionogi) for use as an echocardiographic CM for B (sector) scanning.

Suspensions Containing Microparticles

The first industrial development of echo-enhanced CM, which began about 10 years ago, is based upon suspensions containing microparticles of specially produced galactose particles. This development was successfully concluded with the marketing of SH U 454 (Echovist). A further preparation (SH U 508) is currently being tested.

An identical basic principle underlies both SH U 454 (Echovist) and SH U 508 A. Microparticle granules are suspended shortly before use in specially produced galactose; the suspension is created by shaking these granules in either a galactose solution (Echovist) or in sterile water (SH U 508 A). After the milky-white suspension of microbubbles is injected and makes its passage as a bolus, the blood becomes temporarily echogenic until these acoustic microstructures have been dissolved in the bloodstream [10]. After intravenous injection, SH U 454 (Echovist) dissolves after leaving the right ventricle, as a result of mixing with and being diluted by the blood, before reaching the left ventricle. It is thus suitable for the contrast echocardiographic examination of the right ventricle (and the venous vessel system) by means of B-mode (sector) scan and Doppler. It is also used as an echogenic indicator solution for the sonographic visualization of the patency of the fallopian tubes [12].

SH U 508 A possesses greater intravascular stability than SH U 454, something achieved through a minor galenic change (using physiological fatty acid as an additive). This results in an increase in echogenicity that survives the pulmonary passage after intravenous injection and thus remains, in effect, in the systemic arterial vascular bed. With the bloodstream echogenic during bolus passage, an echogenic contrast imaging of the right and left cardiac cavities in sector scan may be achieved, given adequate dosage; even with a smaller doses, Doppler signal intensity is enhanced.

Areas of Application for Ultrasonographic Contrast Media

Echocardiography

Contrast-enhanced echocardiography of the right ventricle is especially suitable for diagnosing shunts at the atrial or ventricular level and for demonstrating valvular insufficiency. In addition, endocardial definition is improved by echogenic contrast imaging of the right cardiac cavity. Precisely because the echogenic contrast effect of Echovist and other right-ventricle CM is *not* normally supposed to survive pulmonary passage, these CM help in detecting small shunts and especially an open foramen ovale.

The use of CM in colour Doppler echocardiography increases the sensitivity of blood-flow detection. Thus, especially in patients with poor Doppler signal to noise ratios, it can unambiguously image shunts and valvular incompetence where previous tests have been inconclusive [1, 2, 4]. Figure 10.2.1 shows a left to right shunt in an atrial septum defect made visible only by means of Echovist-induced signal intensification.

Contrast-Enhanced Phlebosonography

The contrast imaging of venous return in peripheral and central vessels permits observation of haemodynamics in B mode or an enhancement of Doppler sonographic flow signals. This offers diagnostic advantages: in the exclusion of thromboses and vascular occlusions where plain X-rays are inconclusive, in follow-up in lytic therapy, in the demonstration of venous insufficiency and in the functional assessment of dialysis shunts and vena cava filters [15].

Contrast-Enhanced Hysterosalpingosonography

With the introduction of the first echogenic CM, SH U 454 (Echovist), especially in conjunction with transvaginal examination techniques, it was possible to develop a sonographic alternative to X-ray hysterosalpingography (HSG) [3]. Aside from the diagnosis of uterine anomalies, tubal patency can be demonstrated sonographically by the transcervical administration of Echovist. The advantage of this method over conventional procedures, such as HSG or chromolaparoscopy, consists in the elimination of radiation exposure, allergic CM reactions and/or operative risks. It also allows the patient to observe the examination directly and to witness the results along with the physician. A very detailed description of the examination technique and a discussion of findings and differential may be found in [4].

Clinical studies of tubal patency has resulted in a specificity of 100% and a sensitivity of 88% for contrast-enhanced HSG in comparison to conventional diagnosis (laparoscopy, X-ray HSG) [12]. Contrast-enhanced HSG thus offers a less-invasive screening procedure in fertility investigations.

Preliminary experience with pulsed-wave and colour Doppler vaginal probes show that the addition of Doppler recording can further improve both diagnostic certainty (especially in suspected tubal occlusion) and

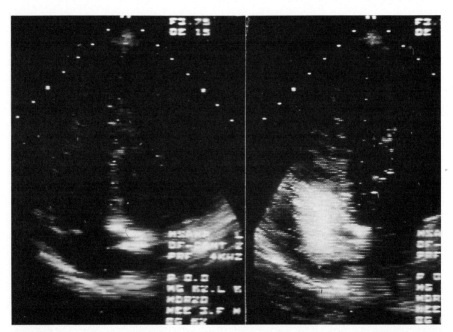

Fig. 10.2.1 a, b. Apical four-chamber image of colour Doppler echocardiography: atrial septal defect with left-right shunt **a** before and **b** after injection of Echovist. *RV*, right ventricle; *RA*, right atrium; *LV*, left ventricle; *LA*, left atrium

visualization [3, 7]. Figure 10.2.2 shows a transvaginal duplex scan. The unhindered tubal flow during CM perturbation is documented here by means of the simultaneously registered Doppler signal.

Additional Areas of Application

The preliminary results of clinical studies of those CM that are stable in the pulmonary capillaries (Albumex, SH U 508 A) have shown that echogenic enhancement in arterial blood after intravenous injection can improve the diagnostic value of the echocardiography of the left ventricle and extend the area of application, especially of vascular Doppler examinations – as has been reported for SH U 508 A. Figure 10.2.3 shows a series of apical four-chamber images during the CM passage of SH U 508 A through both cardiac cavities. Figure 10.2.4 shows a case of mitral insufficiency which was not visible with the conventional colour Doppler technique, but which could be diagnosed on the basis of enhanced Doppler intensity following the intravenous injection of SH U 508 A.

Topics for future studies with SH U 508 A may include: transcranial Doppler sonography; one- and two-dimensional Doppler examinations of central and peripheral vessels, including the trunks of the coronary arteries (per transoesophageal approach); and distinguishing tumours by means of colour Doppler sonography.

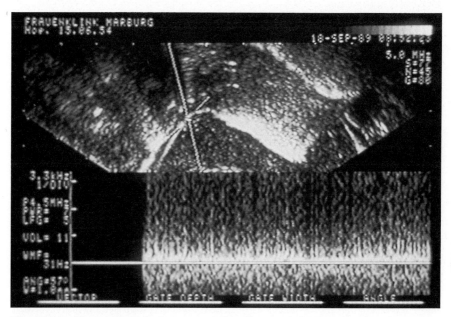

Fig. 10.2.2. Transvaginal duplex sonography: characteristic Doppler signals with the perfusion of Echovist confirms patency of left tubes

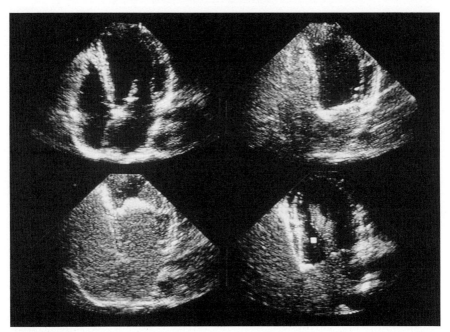

Fig. 10.2.3a–d. Echocardiographic apical four-chamber image **a** before and **b–d** after injection of SH U 508 A. **b** Echogenically marked blood flow in the right cardiac cavities and the inflow into the left atrium after pulmonary passage. **c** First diastolic inflow in the left ventricle. **d** Corresponding end-systolic phase with contrast-enhanced residual blood

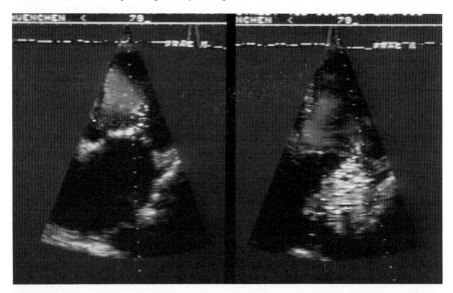

Fig. 10.2.4a, b. Echocardiographic colour Doppler sonography of the left ventricle **a** before and **b** after injection of SH U 508 A. The systolic reflux through the mitral valve in the atrium is only visible after contrast enhancement of the Doppler signal (detection of mitral insufficiency)

References

1. Becher H, Schlief R (1989) Improved sensitivity of color Doppler by SH U 454. Am J Cardiol 64:374–377
2. Becher H, v Bibra H, Glänzer K, Schlief R, Aupperle B, Vetter H (1990) Contrast enhanced colour doppler imaging of left heart chambers. Circulation [Suppl] 82:375
3. Deichert U, Schlief R, van de Sandt M, Juhnke I (1989) Transvaginal hysterosal-pingo-contrast-sonography (Hy-Co-Sy) compared with conventional tubal diagnostics. Hum Reprod 4:418–424
4. Deichert U, Duda V, Schlief R (eds) (1992) Funktionelle Sonographie in der Gynäkologie und Reproduktionsmedizin. Springer, Berlin Heidelberg New York (in press)
5. Feinstein SB, Cheirif J, Ten Cate FJ, Silverman PR, Heidenreich PA, Dick C, Desir RM, Armstrong WF, Quinones MA, Shah PM (1990) Safety and efficacy of a new transpulmonary ultrasound contrast agent: initial multicenter clinical results. J Am Coll Cardiol 16:316–324
6. Gramiak R, Shah PM (1968) Echocardiography of the aortic root. Invest Radiol 3:356
7. Hünecke B, Lindner C, Braendle W (1989) Untersuchung zur Tubenpassage mit der vaginalen gepulsten Kontrastmittel-Doppler-Sonographie. Ultraschall Klin Prax 4:192–198
8. Meltzer RS, Tickner G, Sahines TP, Popp RL (1980) The source of ultrasound contrast effect. J Clin Ultrasound 8:121
9. Reisner AS, Shapiro JR, Amico AF, Meltzer RS (1989) Contrast agents for myocardial perfusion studies. In: Meerbaum S, Meltzer R (eds) Myocardial contrast two-dimensional echocardiography. Kluwer, Dortrecht
10. Schlief R (1988) Echovist©: Physikalisch-pharmakologische Eigenschaften, Ergebnisse klinischer Prüfungen und Anwendungspotential eines neuartigen Ultraschall-Kontrastmittels. Biermann, Münster, pp 163–170 (Jahrbuch der Radiologie)
11. Schlief R (1991) Ultrasound contrast agents. Curr Opin Radiol 3:198–207
12. Schlief R, Deichert U (1991) Hysterosalpingo-contrast-sonography: results of a clinical trial with a novel US contrast medium in 120 patients. Radiology 178:213–215
13. Schlief R, Staks T, Mahler M, Rufer M, Fritzsch T, Seifert W (1990) Successful opacification of the left heart chambers on echocardiographic examination after intravenous injection of a new saccharide based contrast agent. Echocardiography 7:61–64
14. v Bibra H, Hartmann F, Petrick M, Schlief R, Reuner U, Blömer H (1988) Kontrast-Farbdoppler-Echokardiographie. Verbesserte Rechtsherzdiagnostik nach intravenöser Injektion von Echovist. Z Kardiol 78:101–108
15. Vorwerk D, Gehl HB, Schlief R, Nelles A, Günther RW (1990) Dynamische Kontrastmittelgestützte Ultraschallkavographie bei Kavafilterpatienten. Ultraschall Med 11:146–149

Subject Index